<u>Disclaimer</u>

Get your doctors permission making any changes to your diet and exercise program. All individuals should always consult with their doctor before beginning any type of exercise program. The information contained in this book is in no way intended to be used against the advice of a doctor, physician or other qualified health care or medical professional.

The information contained in this book is not to be used as a substitute for any exercise, nutrition or other treatment prescribed by your doctor, physician or other qualified health care or medical professional.

The information in this book is not intended and should not be used to treat, correct, prevent or heal any medical/health related condition.

If you have or suspect you have any illness or other medical/health condition you should always consult with your doctor or health care professional before beginning or making changes to an exercise program.

The author advises the user to know and not exceed his/her limits. Do not perform anything beyond your level of experience, ability, fitness or training level.

Ask your doctor or qualified health care professional to determine which exercises are appropriate for you and for any modifications or exercises to avoid.

The author shall not be held liable or responsible for anyone or anything regarding the information in this book. With all exercise and nutrition programs there are potential risks. The user assumes all risk for injury, loss and/or damage caused or alleged to be caused directly or indirectly by using any information contained in this book.

COPYRIGHT WARNING

i

Table Of Contents

Chapter 1

My Personal Journey
Struggle Leads To Discovery

Chapter 2

Mental and Emotional Stress
The Power Your Thoughts & Emotions Have Over Your Weight

Chapter 3

The TBAR® Cycle
How Your Thoughts Create Your Results

Chapter 4

Getting To Know Your 4 'W's
The Secret To Unstoppable Motivation

Chapter 5

The 'Little-Known' Truth About Nutritional Stress
The Secrets Health & Fitness Experts Aren't Telling You

Chapter 6

The Calorie Reduction Controversy
The Truth You Haven't Been Told About Calories

Chapter 1

<u>My Personal Journey:</u>
Struggle Leads To Discovery

'How could I have gained a pound?' I thought to myself nearly 7 years ago as I stepped on my scale early one Saturday morning.

I was about 4 months into my seemingly impossible mission to re-discover my abs. To complete my mission would require me to lose all 36 pounds hanging from my waist and belly that I had gained during my college years away from home.

I had managed to lose most of the weight but I wanted to lose another 10 pounds.

My exercise routine began with 4 one hour-long workouts each week but had increased significantly because the results would cease after several weeks. In the end I followed a strict exercise regimen that had me on the treadmill, lifting weights or a combination of both 6 days a week for 90 minutes on most days.

I also followed the standard weight loss diet consisting of foods that were low in calories, carbs and fat and high in protein.

During this time, I worked 3 jobs because my wife and I were nearly $50,000 in debt, were barely able to pay the rent on our apartment each month, we were two months behind on most of our bills, had creditors and bill collectors calling our home day and night and had been struggling to conceive our first child for nearly three years with no luck.

I think it's fair to say we were a wee-bit stressed out.

My weight loss had started at a steady pace of 2 pounds per week for the first 4 weeks or so. Soon after it slowed to between a half-pound and one pound per week. Shortly after it was hit or miss where I would lose a pound one week and nothing the next, a half-pound here then nothing there.

I tried every weight loss strategy I could think of to speed up the process like cutting more calories from my diet, increasing the length of my workouts up to 90 minutes on most days and I even increased my workouts from 4 days per week to 6 days per week.

I also began experiencing a lot of unexplained aches and pains I never had before. It started with lower back problems on my left side. Then came the pain in my left hip and my right knee that would show up about half-way into my 90-minute marathon treadmill sessions. I also had pain in my left ankle, a short but excruciating bout of plantar fasciitis and pain in both shoulders following my upper body weight training workouts.

Had I been in my seventies or older I might have expected these problems but at age thirty-two I knew this wasn't good.

I was working so hard and yet struggling to make consistent progress. The culmination was the morning when I woke up to realize that even doing everything I thought was right resulted in me *gaining* back one pound.

I knew something was wrong for weeks but my mind only knew one solution. *More!*

But, I was at the end of my rope where I had nothing more I could realistically do. If what I was doing now wasn't working then going any further certainly wouldn't be the answer. I couldn't fathom the idea of performing 2 hour workouts 6 or worse, 7 days a week.

I had become one of the unfortunates who eat right and exercise regularly yet remain stuck in a weight loss rut where their bodies refuse to change no matter how many calories, carbs or fat they cut out of their diet or how hard, how long or how often they work out. It just didn't make any sense as to why my body suddenly decided to wage an all-out battle against me. I was mentally, emotionally and physically spent.

I was constantly tired, weak and hungry to the point where I had almost non-stop visions of thick, juicy hamburgers and greasy double-pepperoni covered pizzas dancing in my head. I also came to the realization that I could not maintain this rigorous exercise routine much longer. My body felt like it could literally fall apart at any moment.

The Biggest Weight Loss Lie You've Been Led To Believe

In nearly 11 years as a fitness professional I've met and worked with many people who were that former version of me at one time. I've been fortunate to have helped myself and many others achieve their weight loss goals and overcome nagging injuries with a much more manageable diet and exercise routine.

I've also watched those who refused to change their thinking continue to struggle through the painful process of over working themselves with exercise, consuming nutritionally deficient diets and grinding their bodies down to the point of pain and injury all in an effort to fight fat.

Health, fitness and nutrition experts everywhere still rehash the same generalized information about diet and exercise for weight loss. It's all focused on increasing calorie expenditure by eating less and exercising more.

There's only one problem.

Back when I struggled with my weight I started to realize that this information of reducing calories and carbohydrates, consuming more protein and less fat and doing cardio in your *'fat burning zone'* 5 days a week just didn't work for everyone.

I knew this because I tried all of these strategies and while they worked in the beginning the results were short-lived. I also knew many others who were experiencing the same problem.

It seemed the only recommendations from health and fitness experts for continued weight loss was burning more calories. Sure, it seemed logical. After all, if you burn more calories than you consume you create an energy deficit which your body is supposed to account for by using its' own energy reserves leading to increased weight loss.

However, this foundation of logic started to crumble when me and many others including some of my own clients found that increasing the intensity, duration and/or frequency of our workouts did not result in a significant amount of weight loss. In fact, losing weight became even more difficult despite a greater energy deficit.

When exercise alone failed to produce results I learned that simultaneously reducing the number of calories consumed per day even further would significantly contribute to overall caloric expenditure.

The key was the combination of calorie burning exercise with a reduced calorie diet. Together they created what is called a *'calorie deficit'*. According to theory, a larger calorie deficit results in greater weight loss.

After all, if you lost weight on a diet of 1,700 calories a day while exercising 5 days a week for an hour each workout and you reduce your diet to 1,400 calories per day while exercising 6 days a week for an hour each workout you are burning more calories through the increase in exercise and creating a greater calorie deficit through the reduction in calorie consumption.

But, there is a cut-off point where increasing caloric expenditure stops working.

I am not suggesting that calorie reduction does not work at all for weight loss. That would be difficult to do considering how many people have lost weight on reduced calorie diets.

However, if losing weight is simply a matter of *'calories in versus calories out'* then weight loss should continue at the same rate as long as a consistent calorie deficit is maintained.

Unfortunately, this is not the case yet it is the biggest weight loss lie almost everyone is led to believe.

There are two ways to create a calorie deficit through dietary measures: (1) consume less food (2) restrict one or more nutrients.

But, there comes a point where reducing calories and restricting nutrients becomes a source of significant stress on the body that produces a host of negative outcomes.

There are two main problems with calorie reduction and nutrient restriction.

First, reduced calorie and nutrient restricted diets are fundamentally flawed when used as a weight loss strategy and are often a source of increased stress to the body that has negative effects on weight loss.

Second, the reason why these diets work or why they don't is a misunderstood concept that has much less to do with calories than we are being led to believe.

The Story Of Judy

Judy was one of my first personal training clients who had come to me after losing a significant amount of weight through strict dieting and hit a plateau. According to her body mass index that measures body height relative to body weight to determine degree of obesity and body fat percent testing Judy was still considered obese even after losing nearly 100 pounds.

Judy was on a weight loss nutrition program that was anything but healthy. At the time the American College Of Sports Medicine recommended women consume a minimum of 1,200 calories per day for optimum health (In 2005 the U.S. Department Of Agriculture recommended a minimum of 1,800 calories for women of Judy's age). However, Judy's program had her on a diet of just 800 calories per day almost all of which came from vitamin supplements that were not surprisingly sold to her by the company who put her on the nutrition program.

When I suggested her body was undernourished and she needed to consume more food Judy looked at me horrified. Who could blame her? After all, everything we read and hear about tells us we need to eat less to lose weight not more.

However, after much prodding and pleading Judy agreed to try my suggestion of eating more. Up until now, what she was doing wasn't working so she had nothing to lose.

Judy decided to take some time off from her nutrition program but still attended her weekly meetings and within a month of increasing her calories with real food and exercising 3-4 day a week she had lost nearly 10 pounds.

On several occasions, clients of mine who after training for months, remained stuck at their current body weight would then go on vacation for 2 or even 4 weeks at a time and return weighing less than when they left me.

Most of the time they looked more surprised than me admitting they not only strayed from their nutrition plan and enjoyed deserts but did little to no exercise.

I felt stuck in my own personal *Groundhog Day* movie as these clients constantly reminded me how they should go on vacation more.

After seeing so many mixed results where some people lost weight only after increasing their calorie intake and others who exercised 5-7 days per week consuming foods that were low in calories, carbohydrates, fat and sodium but couldn't break past their weight loss plateaus I began to question and research everything I could determined to find an answer.

After more than 10 years of research, trial and error, thousands of hours of education and hands-on personal training sessions working *'in-the-trenches'* with clients one-on-one, semi-privately, in groups and in physical rehabilitation settings I discovered the answer that has allowed me and many of my clients over the years to lose weight, reduce body fat, overcome nagging injuries and improve our health.

The answer lies in the pages of this book.

The 95% Failure Phenomenon

There is a reason for our weight problems but it has little to do the calories we consume, the need for fewer carbohydrates, more protein or less fat.

There is no question that these strategies do work for some however they are limited and the reason why they work is misunderstood.

For example, have you ever wondered why a low-carbohydrate diet works wonders for some while others feel tired, hungry and struggle to lose weight or fail to keep it off?

Or why so many of those who drink diet or zero calorie soft drinks still struggle with their weight?

Or why reduced calorie diets work well in the beginning then creep to an eventual stop no matter how many more calories you cut out?

There is a reason why almost all diets fail, why people can eat healthy and exercise regularly yet fail to reach their weight loss goals and why 95% of those who lose weight gain it back.

Sure, most health and fitness experts and even doctors keep telling us to exercise more and to watch our calories, eat fewer carbs and less fat but why are so many people practicing these strategies and still struggling?

If something is not working shouldn't we question the reason why?

The truth as you're about to discover, is that these and other weight loss strategies are only addressing the *symptoms* yet failing to tackle the *cause* of a much bigger problem.

The Truth About Stress & Your Weight

Stress is a part of our everyday lives. It comes at us in many different ways all the time and is the deciding factor when it comes to losing weight and maintaining weight loss.

Most of us tend to think of stress in an abstract sense such as people who get on our nerves, bosses who stress us out, feeling the pressure of meeting deadlines, paying bills on time or having a heated argument with a loved one.

We seem to know all too well what people, places or events stress us out but one question still looms.

What exactly is stress?

If you're wondering why this is important let me explain. Stress affects us in a number of ways some of which are positive and some of which are negative. There are several negative effects however for the purposes of this book I want to focus on two which are weight gain and weight retention.

As you will discover later in this book, weight gain or the inability to lose weight is the result of taking on more stress then we can handle. So, to lose weight we must effectively understand how to reduce stress. However, in order to reduce stress we first need to know what stress is.

Stress is defined as the following:

'1. Strain; specif., force that strains or deforms 2) emphasis; importance
3) **a) mental or physical tension** b) urgency, pressure, etc. causing this 4) the relative force of utterance given a syllable or word; accent'

Of particular importance is the third definition *'mental or physical tension'* which addresses two important stress factors. However, this definition fails to account for two other equally important stress factors which are *'emotional and nutritional or food stress'.*

There are stressors that we have little to no control over such as those that come from our external environment like air pollution and extreme weather conditions.

Then there are other stressors that we have complete control over. I have identified these stressors as physical, mental, emotional and nutritional.

Most stress reduction strategies only attempt to deal with *negative* stressors.

What they fail to account for are the *positive* stressors because these typically aren't viewed as unhealthy. One of the most popular stress management strategies is exercise because exercise is considered healthy.

But, when you're mentally, emotionally and physically exhausted after a 10 hour work day is it still healthy to go push yourself through a grueling workout at the gym?

In the chapter on physical stress you will learn that exercising too much can put a dead-stop to your weight loss efforts every bit as much as exercising too little.

Contrary to popular belief, stress is not always a bad thing.

In fact, certain amounts of stress are needed for us to lose weight and stay healthy. Problems start to happen as soon as we are pushed beyond our threshold for how much stress we can effectively manage.

Let's look at 3 possible ways to manage our stress levels:

- <u>Raise your stress threshold</u>- Each of us has our own upper limit for handling stress known as our stress threshold. If we stay below our stress threshold we can effectively manage stress and more easily reach our weight loss goals. By raising your stress threshold you are able to handle stress more effectively because it takes more stress to push you over your threshold. This is very effective however the drawback is the amount of time it takes to develop a high enough threshold.

- Use exercise or other constructive activities- This method uses exercise or other physical activities to *'push'* stress out however this does not raise your stress threshold. Instead, stress is managed through elimination. Since this method does not increase your tolerance for stress the control you have over how much stress you can handle is limited.

- Reduce the stressors you control- By becoming consciously aware of your mental, emotional, physical and nutritional stressors you can effectively reduce the amount of stress you experience. This method does not raise your threshold however it may feel as if it does because you are taking on less stress.

As you are about to discover there are many different forms of stress that not only affect our happiness and well being but can keep us from achieving our weight loss goals as well.

How Stress Can Make You Fat

"In a recent article in Psychology Today, "Success...It's Worse Than You Think," medical writer John Carpi discusses the increased sensitivity to stress some of us experience: "...we can become sensitized, or acutely sensitive to stress. Once that happens, even the merest intimation of stress can trigger a cascade of chemical reactions in brain and body that assault us from within."- Harris, 2007.

In his book *'Thresholds Of The Mind'* author Bill Harris describes the concept of stress threshold and how it affects us.

"Thresholds, as I've explained before, are the points where the old system cannot handle further input from the environment, where it cannot dissipate the necessary entropy and, as a result, becomes more chaotic and begins to break down."

It is important to understand that each of us has our own upper limit for handling stress known as our stress threshold. If we stay below our stress threshold we can effectively manage stress and more easily reach our weight loss goals. Every time we experience stress it accumulates and pushes us closer to our threshold. Once our threshold is exceeded our physical and mental abilities to cope with stress become significantly compromised.

As soon as our threshold has been exceeded any further stress elevates our levels of a hormone called cortisol. You may have heard cortisol referred to as the *'stress hormone'*. There is a reason why this is so.

As cortisol levels increase our bodies use more energy from protein and fat. Since most of our protein supply exists within our muscles the body increases the rate of muscle breakdown which increases muscle loss.

Our muscle cells burn most of the energy we use and therefore, as we lose muscle the amount of energy we use is reduced and our metabolism slows down making it more difficult to lose weight and burn fat.

The image below illustrates the stress threshold.

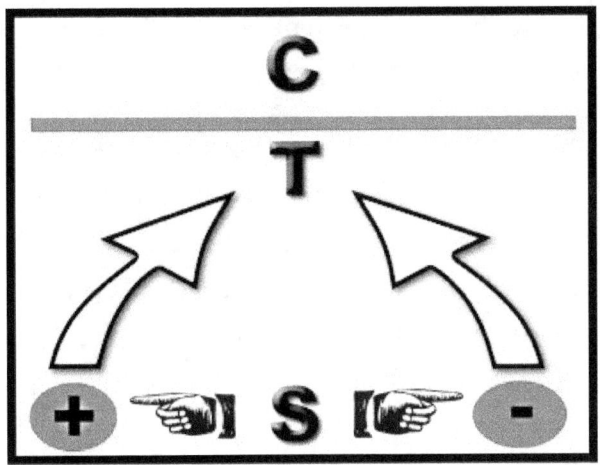

Stress (S) is illustrated at the bottom. Whenever we experience a stressor whether good (+) or bad (-) it accumulates and pushes us closer toward our stress threshold (T). Any further stress beyond our threshold elevates our cortisol levels (C). The long-term effects of elevated cortisol levels include muscle loss, fat storage and weight gain.

How Stress Is Secretly Sabotaging Your Weight

We typically think of stress in general terms such as *'good'* and *'bad'* or *'healthy'* and *'unhealthy'*.

The truth is that your body does not know the difference and therefore it doesn't matter if you are feeling the positive effects following a great workout, if you've been in a car accident or if you're worried about paying the bills for the month; it's still stress as far as your body is concerned.

This is how stress can secretly be sabotaging your weight. Have you ever experienced something similar to the following scenario?

It's Monday morning and you wake up feeling exhausted because you haven't slept well *(physical stress)*. You were restless most of the night because your mind was occupied with the deadline you have to meet for a project at work *(mental stress)*.

So, you fill up your coffee mug to get that morning jolt of caffeine you need to wake up *(food stress)*.

As the morning goes by you're running on a caffeinated high getting all your work completed as fast as you can because you're worried about meeting your deadline *(emotional stress)*.

Then around noon you realize you haven't eaten anything, the caffeine buzz is wearing off and you're feeling a bit weak *(physical stress)*.

Lunchtime comes, you're starving and you gobble down a bigger than normal plate at your favorite local restaurant or café. You return to work but you ate a bit too much and now feel sluggish so you grab another cup of coffee and off you go for the rest of the day *(more food stress)*.

As your workday is coming to an end you're feeling physically and mentally exhausted and you are looking forward to getting home for some much needed rest and relaxation *(more physical, mental and emotional stress)*.

But, you suddenly remember your exercise class is tonight and you really need to lose those 15 pounds you've been struggling with. You reluctantly drag yourself into the gym and manage to get through the workout *(even more physical stress)*.

You return home wiped out and starving once again (after all you haven't eaten since lunch) and chomp down a big dinner, crash on the sofa and zone out watching television until bedtime *(even more food stress)*.

As crazy as it seems, these are elements of a typical work day for so many people who consistently operate beyond their stress threshold. Stress plays the ultimate role in determining whether or not you lose weight.

It does not matter if the stress is good or bad because your body cannot tell the difference. If you keep piling stress onto a system that's overwhelmed with stress that system will eventually break down and you will find it extremely difficult to lose weight and keep it off.

"Our body has no way of differentiating a physical stress from an emotional, mental or a spiritual stress. To the nervous system and hormonal system, it doesn't matter whether you've just had a car accident, are going through a divorce, are under the pressure of too many deadlines at work, or even just won $100,000,000 in the lottery! Your hormonal and nervous systems react the same way – it's just stress." -Chek

The Stress Response Systems

To gain a better understanding of how your body responds to stress let's take a look at the 2 key stress response systems of the human body.

The nervous system is the body's control center. You can think of it as your body's internal communication network. In order for your body to move, muscles must contract. Muscles contract when given the nerve impulse from the brain. The communication of the nerve impulse from the brain is carried to the muscles through the nervous system.

The nervous system is divided into 2 parts: the central nervous system and the peripheral nervous system. For our purposes we will focus on the peripheral nervous system.

The peripheral nervous system is also divided into 2 parts: somatic and autonomic.

The autonomic nervous system is further divided into 2 branches: the sympathetic and parasympathetic nervous systems. It is these two nervous system branches that respond to stress and determine whether or not you lose weight.

The NOT-SO Sympathetic Nervous System

The sympathetic nervous system (SNS) is your body's response to stress.

Activation of the SNS produces a *'fight-or-flight'* response which you've experienced if you've ever been in a situation that caused you extreme fear of danger.

These are situations where people are capable of performing almost superhuman feats of strength such as the story of a mother who rescued her young boy from being pinned underneath an automobile by lifting one side of the car off of the ground.

Once activated the SNS increases production of the stress hormones epinephrine, nor epinephrine and cortisol. You may not be familiar with the first two but chances are you have heard of cortisol. Cortisol is often referred to as the *'stress hormone'* and for good reason.

The Devastating Effects Of Stress

When blood glucose (a.k.a blood sugar) levels drop your body activates a stress response by releasing the hormone cortisol into the bloodstream.

When blood glucose levels fall too low cortisol levels rise in an attempt to help raise your blood glucose levels back to normal. Part of cortisol's role is to conserve blood glucose which it does by triggering the breakdown and release of protein from muscle tissue and fat from fat cells.

Your body can prioritize whether to use more protein or fat as an energy source depending on how much of an energy deficient state you are in at the time.

The bigger the energy deficit becomes the more the body breaks down muscle tissue and here's why...

...Muscles use more energy versus fat and therefore when your body is trying to conserve energy it will choose to *'get rid of'* the most energy costing material which is muscle tissue. In other words, muscle loss slows down your metabolism making it harder to lose weight and easier to gain weight.

Here's something else to think about.

Your heart is also a muscle. You've heard of the term *'stress kills'* right? This is just one of many ways in which this can happen.

The Truth About Diets & Your Metabolism

Most of the energy we burn occurs inside our muscle cells. Groups of individual muscle cells that are tightly bound together make up what we call our muscles.

Carbohydrates, protein and fats are transported to our muscles and extracted into our muscle cells where they are used to produce the energy we need to move, breathe and stay alive. The more muscle you have the more energy you burn and the faster your metabolism is. The less muscle you have the less energy you burn and the slower your metabolism is.

Muscle loss is a recipe for disaster when you're trying to lose weight because your muscles are essentially your metabolism and the more muscle you lose the slower your metabolism becomes making it harder to keep off the weight you've already lost let alone lose more weight.

Muscle loss is one reason why so many dieters who lose a lot of weight in the beginning on very low calorie or nutrient restricted diets are unable to keep the weight off.

It's also why most not only gain back the weight they lost but a few extra pounds. This happens because with a slower metabolism they are no longer burning the same amount of energy as they were before the diet and even though they return to their *'normal'* pre-diet intake consisting of roughly the same amount of food on average, this puts them in an energy surplus where they are consuming more food energy than their bodies can use leading to the extra weight gain.

My wife Veronica had battled her weight most of her life. She had tried many different diets involving calorie or nutrient restriction or taking pills that would decrease her appetite making her eat less and lose weight. Several times she lost quite a bit of weight on these diets but would ultimately hit a plateau where her weight wouldn't budge. She found herself feeling tired, weak and hungry until she couldn't ignore the signals her body was giving her to eat.

She eventually would come off the diets or the pills because they were too restrictive to stick with and each time she not only gained back all the weight she lost but a few extra pounds along with it.

Over the years she had progressively gained over 30 pounds and to top it off had chronic knee and lower back pain.

Veronica had lost a significant amount of muscle from all the dieting that caused her metabolism to become slower after each diet.

Today she is 19 years older and 45 pounds lighter despite going through pregnancy 4 years ago. She has not resorted to fad diets or pills in over 15 years, she exercises regularly and eats more now than she did during her 20's and she maintains her new body without counting calories, weighing foods or tracking points. She simply follows the 14 'P's of stress free nutrition that I'll be sharing with you a bit later in this book.

And, it's never too late. Over the past 11 years I've worked with people in their 30's, 40's, 50's and even in their 60's who have gone on to lose weight, eliminate nagging injuries and reclaim their health.

What Your Sweet Cravings Really Mean

Glucose is a simple sugar that is made when carbohydrates are broken down in the body. Glucose is the body's preferred energy source and is often referred to as *'blood sugar'*. Chains of glucose called glycogen are stored primarily in your muscles and minimally in your liver.

When you constantly skip meals or an hour or two after eating foods that quickly convert to sugar your blood glucose levels can take a nose-dive and your SNS responds by releasing cortisol. Cortisol triggers the release of glycogen from the liver into the bloodstream to quickly raise your blood glucose levels.

However, as this is happening, most people feel weak, shaky or low on energy which many refer to as having *'low blood sugar'*. This experience is accompanied by intense cravings for sugary foods or drinks which often results in the consumption of sweets, soda or other sugar-loaded snacks.

When combined with the glycogen released from the liver this creates a massive insulin surge similar to a pinball machine screaming *'full-tilt!'*

Insulin is a hormone your body produces to lower your blood glucose levels. The higher your blood glucose levels are the more insulin your body produces. Insulin lowers blood glucose levels by storing glucose, protein and fat. Insulin plays a much needed role within the body however when your blood glucose levels are constantly elevated and your body keeps releasing large amounts of insulin the side effect is fat storage.

↑ CORTISOL = ↑ BLOOD GLUCOSE = ↑ INSULIN = FAT STORAGE

Unfortunately, this creates a constant roller coaster ride where blood glucose levels go way up and come crashing down leading to intense cravings for sweets, overeating, weight gain and the accumulation of body fat.

Your Body's Secret Trigger For Fat Storage

Food isn't the only thing that triggers fat storage. When your stress levels exceed your threshold you enter what can be described as a **'sympathetic nervous system (SNS) dominant state'**.

This is your body's secret trigger for fat storage and here's why...

...If you constantly remain in a SNS dominant state this is described as *'catabolic'* which basically means *'breaking down'*. So, dominance of the SNS results in an increase in the breakdown and use of muscle tissue for energy which ultimately slows down the metabolism.

The long-term effects of SNS dominance are indigestion, constipation, chronic fatigue, weight gain, immune system suppression and increased vulnerability to sickness and disease.

We live in a fast-paced world where most people are stressed out 24 hours a day, 7 days a week and go about their days in a SNS dominant state like they're stuck in a never-ending Nascar race.

They have no energy and rely on caffeine and sugar-filled foods to get them through the day. They get sick or have nagging aches and pains and depend heavily on over-the-counter or prescription medications. They become overweight and believe that the next *'miracle weight loss pill'* or fad diet will solve the problem only to realize the only weight they really lost was the dollars from their wallets.

Most people are overwhelmed by stress and constantly pushed over their threshold. Then they try to *'fix'* the symptoms by trying all kinds of fad diets, workouts that are too hard, too long or too often, exercises to tone this, trim that, slim down and shape up that further push their SNS through the roof only to end up frustrated and burned out when these *'remedies'* fail to provide a solution.

You don't get an alcoholic to quit drinking by giving him more alcohol. Nor will you decrease an SNS dominant state by doing the very things that trigger it.

Brief periods of SNS activity are beneficial and healthy. Problems occur when the SNS becomes the dominant branch of the nervous system. As long as the SNS stays within your threshold for stress you have balance with the parasympathetic nervous system (PNS) which is your body's recovery or rebuilding system.

Your Body's Built-In Stress Relief System

The parasympathetic nervous system (PNS) is your body's stress relief system.

The PNS increases anabolic hormones (growth hormone, testosterone, DHEA) that support tissue repair, growth and maintenance. Peak PNS activity occurs during sleep and periods of rest or inactivity.

However, over activation of the PNS can result in low energy levels, difficulty managing blood sugar levels, chronic aches and pains, muscle loss, weight gain, constipation, disease, heart and circulatory problems and emotional imbalance due to lack of movement.

The image below illustrates the role of the SNS and PNS in response to stress. The SNS dominant zone at the top represents a stress level that's too high (over threshold). The PNS dominant zone at the bottom represents a stress level that's too low. The POWER zone in the middle represents balance of all 4 stressors.

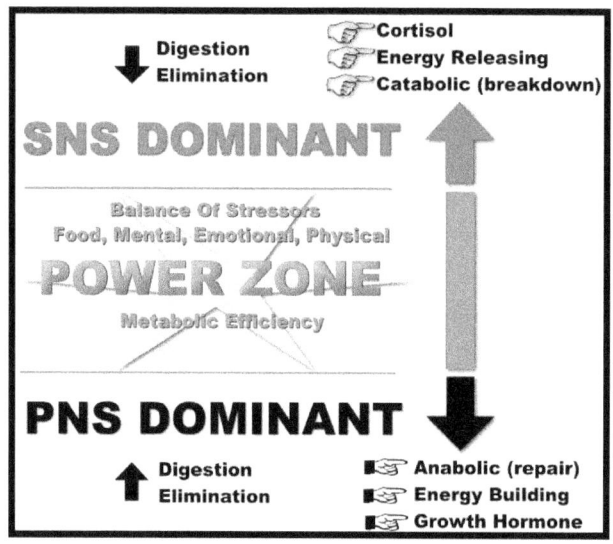

Too much stress results in SNS dominance, muscle breakdown, decreased recovery, poor digestion and increased fat storage. Too little stress results in PNS dominance which can be good if your body is overworked and needs some down time. However, a PNS dominant state can be detrimental toward weight loss and optimum health due to the lack of energy movement throughout the body.

A New Vision For You

We live in a nation where the majority of people feel disempowered, frustrated, confused and have lost hope of ever achieving their weight loss goals. Others are stuck dealing with chronic aches and pains that doctors, medicine and physical rehabilitation are unable to resolve. Since you are reading this book you are likely a part of this majority.

Maybe you *really* want to lose 25 pounds or more but after one or more failed attempts you tell yourself you'll be just as happy losing 10 pounds.

Maybe you're dealing with a nagging injury that's forced you to limit or avoid your favorite recreational sports activities and you've accepted that this is what happens when you get older.

Whatever it is I want to make one point crystal clear.

Your struggles are not your fault. You simply have done the best you could based on the information you have available. Unfortunately, anyone anywhere in the world can provide information on just about anything. If you don't believe me then Google the term *'weight loss'* and see how many results turn up. <u>As I write this there are 323 million!</u>

We're drowning in a sea of information yet struggling to figure out where to begin. The overwhelming amount of information available makes it nearly impossible to distinguish good information from misinformation.

It is not your fault if the *'Super Celebrity Magic Makeover Diet'* that's guaranteed to make you lose so much weight you'll become invisible didn't work for you. You have not failed your diet and exercise program. Your diet and exercise program have failed you.

The good news is that I am here to provide the information that's right for you so you can finally achieve your weight loss goals and get your life back on track.

The first thing is to understand that the only way you are ever going to end your struggles with your weight is by addressing the root cause of the problem which is stress.

By using the information in this book you will discover the last 4 stress reducing secrets you'll ever need to look, feel and move your best. Although, there are only 4 do not dismiss them as unimportant.

Each one plays a significant role in determining whether or not you lose weight, and keep it off.

This is the first book of its kind that addresses the 4 stress factors as the true cause of weight problems and provides some simple yet highly effective stress reducing solutions that can easily be applied to win the fight against fat once and for all.

In this book you will learn about the devastating effects of mental stress and how your thoughts can and do sabotage your efforts to lose weight without you even realizing it.

I will also reveal the truth about emotional stress and how your emotions can be your best friend or your worst enemy when it comes to losing weight.

You will also understand the hidden nutritional stressors most health and fitness experts aren't telling you about and why low-calorie diets, nutrient restriction and many so-called *'healthy'* foods recommended by most health and fitness experts are keeping you from reaching your weight loss goals.

And, finally there is physical stress; why your body responds well to exercise some of the time and fights tooth and nail against it at other times and what you can do about it so losing weight is no longer a battle of wills between you and your body.

So, buckle up and get ready...

...Your journey toward achieving your ideal weight and enjoying vibrant health is about to begin!

Chapter 2

Mental and Emotional Stress:
The Power Your Thoughts and Emotions Have Over Your Weight

There is an ongoing debate about which is most important when it comes to losing weight: diet or exercise.

While both have significant merits I disagree that either one is the *most important* component for successful weight loss, body fat reduction and vibrant health.

After all, diet and exercise fail to explain why so many people:

- Do not believe they can achieve their weight loss and fitness goals

- Know they need to eat better and exercise more but still fail to do so

- Start on a weight loss program only to quit within the first few months

- Experience some success then sabotage themselves for no apparent reason

- Cannot find the motivation to lose weight they desperately want to lose

Over the last 11 years as a fitness professional and applying principles of personal achievement, success and motivation to help my clients overcome the mental and physical obstacles in order to achieve their goals I have come to understand that neither the best diet nor the best exercise program will amount to much without first addressing the most powerful component...

...your mind!

Although this is the most in-depth part of this book it's also the most important.

Most weight loss programs deal with diet and exercise yet fail to establish the proper mental and emotional states needed for long-term success.

Mental and emotional stress go hand-in-hand and are so powerful that you will fail to get the results you want even with the most effective diet and exercise program money can buy if your mental and emotional states are not properly programmed for success.

In this chapter, you will understand how your thoughts and emotions affect your physiology and can be your best friend or worst enemy when it comes to losing weight.

This chapter is as much about doing as it is about learning. Reading the information will give you knowledge but knowledge by itself is not enough to change your body.

Applied knowledge is what gets results.

For this reason there are '*action steps*' at specific points in the next few chapters. The action steps are designed to help you create the proper mindset and develop unstoppable motivation to achieve your goals.

Please be sure to do each action step.

You Are What You ~~Eat~~ Think

We often think of stress as related only to things like our job such as when we have deadlines and demands to meet, finances such as paying the mortgage or bills for the month, relationships such as arguments with loved ones or being preoccupied with too much to do and not enough time.

Yet, when it comes to weight loss we often fail to realize the extent to which mental stress can affect our ability to achieve our goals.

Let's say you're frustrated because you're not losing weight and you can't stand the way your body looks. Every time you look at yourself in the mirror you don't have to say anything because those thoughts start running through your head.

In fact, you have plenty of *'evidence'* to support your thoughts because you've tried just about every diet and exercise routine without any real success.

Now, let's see an example of how this plays itself out.

It's Friday night and you're out with a group of friends or family members at your favorite restaurant and you're skimming over the menu. Suddenly, you have a dilemma on your hands. A tiny little angel appears on your left shoulder reminding you of the healthy food options that will support your weight loss goals. Then on your right shoulder a tiny little devil appears tempting you to go for the *'oh-so-yummy-for-your-tummy'* decadent dishes that you know will ruin your weight loss efforts.

You're stuck at a fork in the road as the waitress begins taking orders from your table. Someone orders the *'Mouth-Watering Mega-Melt Bacon Burger'*, another person orders the *'Terrific Taco Trio'*, the person next to you chooses the *'Pepperoni Pizzazz Pizza'* and now it's your turn to order. You know what you need to do but those thoughts start running through your head:

'My diet isn't working anyway'

'I deserve to enjoy myself'

'I can't lose weight so what's the use'

'I'll eat what I want tonight and just workout extra hard tomorrow'

The angel on your left disappears while the devil on your right stands there grinning as you order the *'Mile-High Pile O'Pasta with the Endless Basket Of Breadsticks'*.

You wake up the next morning and step on the scale and notice your bodyweight hasn't changed. Or perhaps it's gone up a bit. Either way you feel the frustration brewing inside as you tell yourself

'See, I can't lose weight!'

It's this pattern that repeats itself week after week, month after month and quite possibly year after year which reinforces the same thought that you cannot lose weight.

And, it's not only mental stress that's the problem.

The Powerful Influence Of E (nergy In) Motion

The thoughts we have lead to feelings or what we call *emotions* which have a powerful influence on our weight and health.

Emotions are strong, powerful feelings that affect us on a deep, cellular level.

'Your energies are, in fact, so distinctive, and they so potently regulate your physical body, that you begin to look like your energy body just as surely as two people who share a life for fifty years sometimes begin to resemble each other. As your energy field pulses through your body, it gradually adds its complexion to the physical structure that was determined by your genes. Matter follows energy.' –Eden, 1998.

Our cells contain genetic information called 'DNA'. Our DNA defines how our bodies are made up. So, our bodies look and function according to how they are programmed by our DNA. But, unlike what we previously thought, our DNA is not necessarily set in stone.

In the book *The Divine Matrix*, author Gregg Braden explains a study in the 1990's performed by the Institute of HeartMath. In 1991 HeartMath was formed for the specific purpose of exploring the power human feelings have over the body and the role those emotions play in our world.

Between 1992 and 1995 HeartMath researchers tested the effects of human emotion on DNA by isolating human DNA in a glass beaker and then exposing it to a powerful form of feeling known as *coherent emotion*. They used special techniques that analyze DNA both chemically and visually so they could detect any changes that occurred.

They found unmistakable implications that human emotion alone changed the shape of the DNA by creating precise feelings in the participants' bodies!

Different emotional states trigger the production of chemical messengers called *hormones* that interact with and influence the function of specific cells within your body.

Most people believe it's the balance of calories in and out that determines whether or not they lose weight when in reality this plays only a small part. It's our **hormones** that control our metabolism and play the biggest role in weight loss and body fat reduction.

And, since your hormones are influenced by your emotional state this means that your emotions can and do determine whether or not you lose weight.

"In May 2004, a group of scientists at Italy's University of Turin Medical School conducted an unprecedented study investigating the power of belief to heal in a medical situation. It began with administering drugs that mimic dopamine and relieve patients' symptoms. It's important to note here that the drugs have a short life span in the body and their effects last only about 60 minutes. As they wear off, the symptoms return. Twenty-four hours later, the patients under-went a medical procedure where they believed that they would receive a substance to restore their brain chemistry to normal levels. In reality, however,

they were given a simple saline solution that should have had no effect on their condition.

Following the procedure, electronic scans of the patients' brains showed something that's nothing short of a miracle. Their brain cells had responded to the procedure as if they'd been given the drug that originally eased their symptoms. Commenting on the remarkable nature of the study, the team's leader, Fabrizio Benedetti, stated, "It's the first time we've seen it [the effect] at the single neuron level."' The University of Turin findings supported studies that had been conducted earlier by a team at the University of British Columbia in Vancouver. In that investigation, it was reported that placebos could actually raise the brain levels of dopamine in the patients who receive them..."-Braden, 2008.

Not only is the old saying *'you are what you eat'* true but apparently you are what you think as well.

Negative emotional states can lead to problems such as fear, worry, anxiety, depression; feeling overwhelmed and can lead to other problems such as poor mental and physical performance, overeating and weight gain.

You have experienced the amazing power of your emotions first-hand if you've ever woken up from an intense dream, felt your heart racing and you were breathing as if you just ran a marathon only to realize it was just a dream and the events that took place only happened in your mind. But, your body responded just as if they were really happening.

Emotional stress activates the sympathetic nervous system in a fight-or-flight response which:

- Increases your breathing and heart rate to make more oxygen and nutrients available to your muscles
- Diverts the bulk of your blood supply to your large muscles groups to run or fight
- Shuts down digestion in order to divert blood, nutrients, and oxygen to working muscles
- Triggers the release of glucose into the bloodstream from your liver which requires insulin to metabolize and shuts down fat loss
- Stimulates your adrenal glands to release the stress hormones epinephrine and norepinephrine
- Stimulates the release of cortisol which promotes fat storage

As you can see, when you are chronically stressed out on an emotional level your body undergoes powerful hormonal changes that make it nearly impossible to lose weight and reduce body fat.

Another problem with excessive stress is muscle tension. When our muscles contract they produce tension in order to maintain posture, move our bodies and support and protect our vital organs. However, excessive muscle tension can lead to muscle imbalances and result in negative effects such as headaches, poor posture and joint alignment, physical aches and pains, chronic fatigue, poor endurance, reduced strength, restricted blood and energy flow, organ dysfunction, sickness and disease.

Excessive muscular tension can also wreak havoc on your efforts to lose body fat. To lose fat oxygen and nutrients including fatty acids must be transported through the bloodstream to your muscle cells where they are burned as energy.

However, excessive muscle tension decreases the diameter of the blood vessels restricting the flow of blood, oxygen, fatty acids and other nutrients to the muscle cells. This results in a decrease in energy availability leading to chronic fatigue, poor muscular and cardiovascular endurance, losses in strength and decreased fat loss.

While a certain amount of stress is needed and beneficial for us too much stress in any form can have devastating effects on both your weight and health.

So, you now know the extent to which your emotional states can impact your ability to lose weight. I am not saying that any and every single negative emotion will keep you from losing weight. Negative emotions are perfectly normal. The problems that occur are the result of being stuck in a constant cycle of negative emotional states.

Your emotions are triggered by your thoughts and therefore changing your emotional state begins with changing your thoughts.

This is a critical element that weight loss diets and exercise programs fail to address. Constant negative thoughts result in a vicious mental cycle that is, in my experience, the main reason why most people struggle to lose weight and keep it off. I call this the TBAR® Cycle which stands for:

THOUGHTS => BELIEFS => ACTIONS => RESULTS

Let's take a look at the TBAR® Cycle and the effects it can have on your weight...

Chapter 3

The TBAR Cycle:
How Your Thoughts Create Your Results

Emotions are rooted within the TBAR® Cycle resulting from a constant pattern of thoughts as you will see. The TBAR® Cycle begins with thoughts that create your beliefs. Those beliefs then influence your actions. The actions you take produce your results. And, the results you get reinforce your thoughts.

Let's look a bit deeper into the TBAR® Cycle to gain a better understanding of how it all plays out:

Thoughts

Your thoughts are much more powerful than you may realize. Many of the thoughts we have are active beyond our conscious awareness and operate on auto-pilot. Thoughts are ideas that are the seeds from which beliefs grow. When a thought is expressed enough a belief is created.

For example, the thought *'I can't lose weight'* begins as an idea or a concept that expresses itself over and over until it becomes a belief.

Beliefs

A belief is a conviction that a thought is true. It doesn't matter if the issue in question is, in reality, true or not. It's the *conviction* that makes it real for the person.

This is why two people can watch a movie or witness an event yet have completely different perspectives about what happened.

Our minds operate in a manner similar to a computerized e-mail system. When you check your e-mail you probably notice that some e-mail makes it directly to your inbox while some goes directly into your junk folder. This happens automatically without you doing anything.

Why does this happen?

It's because your e-mail system automatically processes the incoming e-mail and filters out what it considers is not useful. E-mail systems run on auto-pilot and our minds operate in a similar manner *(unless we develop the conscious awareness to do otherwise).*

In reality, our eyes do not actually *'see'* they merely take in light from our world. It is our brain that takes this information coming in through our eyes and edits it in a way that makes sense to us based on our beliefs and worldview.

In other words, our brain is what actually *'sees'* not our eyes.

It has been suggested that we only see about 50% of the information that our eyes pick up and our brain processes the other 50% automatically according to our beliefs and without us even realizing it. Therefore, a large portion of what we see is really determined by what we believe is true. The old saying *'I'll believe it when I see it'* is actually backwards.

The reality is we see what we believe.

If you believe strongly enough that you cannot lose weight, that eating right doesn't work for you, that exercise works for everyone else but you or something similar you will find the evidence to support your beliefs all around you even though it may not be true because your brain will automatically *'delete'* any information that goes against your beliefs.

Remember, a belief is nothing more than a conviction and therefore your beliefs are your own convictions that your thoughts or worldview is true regardless of whether it is or is not. So, permanent weight loss doesn't begin with diet and exercise because you could have the best program money could buy and still fail to ever reach your weight loss goal if you believe that you cannot lose weight.

Your Results Are A Reflection Of Your Beliefs

About 10 years ago a man named Larry came to me for personal training and during our consultation when I asked him what his fitness goals were he looked at me completely blank. He sat quiet for about 20 seconds then said *"I don't know"*.

I asked him why he wanted personal training and he mentioned how he wanted to get in better shape but when I asked him what *'better shape'* meant to him he again replied *"I don't know"*.

I knew that without a specific goal to focus on Larry would stand very little chance for getting in *'better shape'* because he didn't know what the end result looked like for him.

"What goals do most people work on with you?" Larry asked.

"They usually want to lose weight, gain muscle, overcome nagging injuries or improve their performance in a particular sport." I replied.

"I guess I'd like to lose some weight and gain muscle." Larry said.

"Ok, if you had to pick one of those which is most important to you" I asked.

Larry sat silent while thinking.

"Probably gaining muscle" he answered.

With a goal in mind I began working with Larry. I trained him 2-3 days per week depending on his work schedule, gave him independent workouts to do on certain days or if he had to leave town on travel and advised him on the nutritional changes he would need to make in order to achieve his goal.

But, Larry was extremely inconsistent with his workouts and his nutrition. In fact, after most of our training sessions he would go across the street to a well-known fast food franchise and order a couple of chicken burritos and other items that he knew he would not support his goal.

In fact, he ate some sort of fast food almost every day for lunch and dinner.

When I asked him why he kept failing to make the changes necessary to support his fitness goal he would laugh it off, make jokes or speak negatively about himself.

I soon realized the problem with Larry was two-fold.

One problem was that he didn't really see himself as lean and more muscular. He simply chose a goal that sounded good to him at the time but he did not believe that he would really achieve it.

The other problem was that deep down Larry did not know what he wanted from his fitness program. He wanted to get in better shape but had no clear idea of what that actually meant to him. The idea of gaining muscle wasn't enough to keep him motivated.

So, even if Larry had gotten into better shape he likely wouldn't have realized it because he wasn't clear about what being in shape looked like to him.

You can't hit a target if you don't know what you're aiming at.

This is part of what I call knowing your 4-W's that you will learn in a bit.

This is also what weight loss and diet programs completely overlook and fail to address and why 95% of those who lose weight eventually gain it all back.

Sure you could point out all the reasons that cause people like Larry to fall of their diet program or fail to stay consistent with their exercise routine but in looking at the underlying issues as to **WHY** this happens, especially when they have experienced success, there are subconscious beliefs at work behind the scenes undermining even their best efforts.

These subconscious beliefs are typically disguised as not having the time to exercise, life getting too busy, forgetting to go shopping or to prepare healthy meals and eating junk food, loss of motivation, making poor food choices, overeating, waiting for the right time to start again, and many other *'reasons'*.

Just like in the previous restaurant example, having unsupportive beliefs will cause you to sabotage yourself without you even realizing it! It may even seem as if forces beyond your control are responsible when, in fact, they are not. If you're going to reach your weight loss goals you're going to need to change your thoughts and beliefs to those that support the achievement of your goals which I will show you how to do in just a bit.

But, first let's look at the third part of the TBAR® Cycle.

Actions

Action is where the proverbial *'rubber meets the road'*. It is the process of moving beyond thinking and into actual doing.

All of the positive thinking you can muster will do nothing to produce the results you want without taking action.

Every action you take produces a result whether it's good or bad.

This means that YOU are entirely responsible for the results you have or have not achieved because you have produced these results intentionally or unintentionally by the actions you have or have not taken.

This might seem pretty deflating right now and you might be blaming yourself or you might find that previous sentence offensive.

Either way the good news is that you can start producing the results you want right now because YOU create your results.

For example, if you justify your lack of progress by telling yourself that you don't have the time to exercise think about it. Don't you have the time somewhere in your day to exercise?

I am willing to bet that if your doctor told you that your life depended on you finding 20-30 minutes a day to exercise you'd be able to do so.

You might try any of the following:

- Getting up 30 minutes earlier to exercise

- Cutting out 20 minutes of television in the evening to exercise

- Exercising on your lunch break

- Exercising for 15 minutes in the morning and 15 minutes in the evening

Do you see how you can find the time to exercise somewhere in your day?

Where in your day can you find the time to exercise?

Action Step: **Get a sheet of paper and write down all of the ways you can find at least 20 minutes a day to exercise. Make 2 copies and post a copy of this sheet somewhere you will see it every day.**

Also, keep a copy with you at all times and read it several times throughout your day as a reminder.

As the saying goes *'out of sight, out of mind'*.

This may seem a bit silly but it will help you create new supportive exercise habits by taking action. And, by consistently taking action you are taking the necessary steps toward creating the results you want.

If you tell yourself that this won't work or that you don't need to do this simple exercise then understand that this is your old way of thinking or what I call your *'Self-Sabotage Mechanism'* (SSM) that is trying to keep you right where you are now.

If you continue to do what you've always done up until now you will only get the results you've always got up until now. If you want better results you need to take a different approach.

Are you willing to take this simple approach to start creating the results you want?

Results

Results are the outcomes we get based upon our actions. Every action you take produces a result whether it's one you want or one you do not want.

Results are extremely powerful because they reinforce your thoughts and as you now know, the entire TBAR® Cycle begins with your thoughts.

Positive thoughts create positive beliefs. Positive beliefs create positive actions. Positive actions create positive results. Positive results reinforce positive thoughts.

However, the opposite also holds true.

If you've been unable to achieve and maintain your weight loss goals it's important to understand that somewhere within you negative thoughts are operating and chances are that these thoughts are running beneath your conscious awareness. In other words, they are happening automatically.

In order to change your results you need to take positive actions that will produce the results you desire. But, in order to take those actions you need to adopt beliefs that support taking those positive actions. And, in order to adopt supportive beliefs you need to change your thoughts from negative to positive.

Unfortunately, it's not as easy as it sounds now is it?

You can say all the positive things in the world but if you don't truly believe them in your heart it really doesn't matter because your SSM will find ways to ruin your efforts.

Your subconscious mind is very much like the hard drive on your computer in that it's been operating automatically beyond your conscious awareness according to how it has been *'programmed'*.

Your subconscious programming is based on many different things such as your own experiences, things your parents said to you, their view of the world, teachers, relatives, friends and others who have influenced you long ago perhaps during your early childhood years.

Take a minute and think about a belief you have and try to identify where you picked it up. Who, what or where did that belief come from?

Many of the beliefs we have were inherited and are not ones we consciously chose.

Now, think of a negative belief you have about your body or your weight and try to identify where that belief really came from.

- Was it based on a parent, sibling or friend who told you that you can't lose weight or you don't have the body type to look the way you want or something similar?

- Was it based on one negative experience you had with a diet or exercise routine that led you to believe that you cannot lose weight?

- Perhaps you failed to achieve the results you wanted from a diet or workout routine that led you to believe that ALL diets and exercise routines don't work.

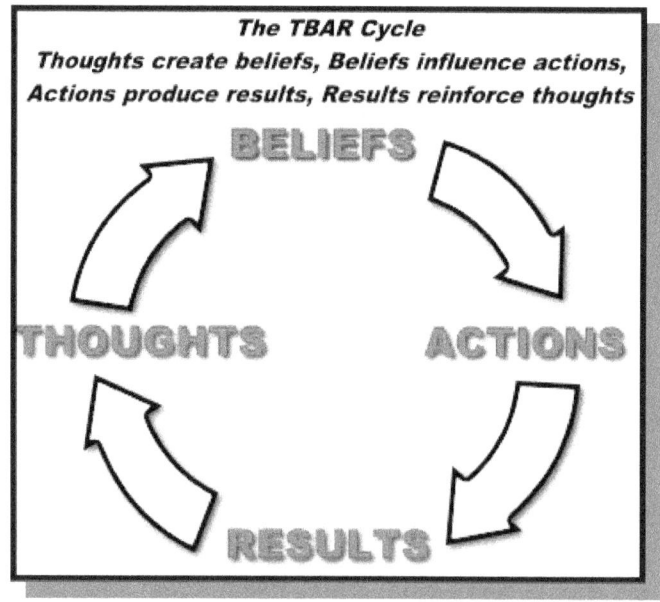

The TBAR Cycle
Thoughts create beliefs, Beliefs influence actions,
Actions produce results, Results reinforce thoughts

BELIEFS

THOUGHTS   ACTIONS

RESULTS

All of the negative beliefs that you have about your body or losing weight creates mental stress and as you can see, this kind of mental stress will keep you from ever achieving your weight loss goals.

The question now is what can you do about it?

The obvious answer is to simply decrease the negative mental and subsequent emotional stress you're creating by changing your negative beliefs. However, changing negative beliefs requires some positive action on your part.

This is why it's important to think **positive thoughts**. These positive thoughts are your affirmations that will help you stay focused on achieving your weight loss goals.

Now, if this sounds like some lame law of attraction voodoo I can assure you it's not.

You might be thinking that something so simple is just plain silly and will never work. I am not asking you to automatically believe it will work however I am asking that you simply put aside your disbelief for the time being.

Look at it this way. Your old ways of thinking and believing have led you to the actions you've taken which have created your results to this point and obviously are not serving you.

Remember your SSM.

You and ONLY you have the power to choose your thoughts and what you believe so why not choose ones that support you and your goals? Besides, what do you have to lose?

Fair enough?

Good.

Now, let's do a simple exercise that will create new positive thoughts that will eventually become beliefs that will support you and put an end to your SSM once and for all.

Think of those negative thoughts you have every time you look at yourself in the mirror, when you step on the scale and haven't lost weight, when you've gained weight, when you've felt guilty about eating *'bad'* food, when you look at your stomach, hips, butt, thighs, waist or arms, when you look at your *'skinny'* clothes in the closet and feel depressed about not being able to fit in them, when you look in your favorite magazines and see models who have the body you desire.

Recall the negative things you say to your friends, family or co-workers about your weight or your body.

Next, you'll need a sheet of paper to write on. Trying to do this exercise in your head will not work. You need to put pen to paper and have it right there in front of you in plain view.

Action Step: **On a sheet of paper list 5-10 negative thoughts or beliefs you have about your body (leave one line of space between each):**

Example: "I'll never lose weight"

Look at your list of negative thoughts or beliefs and read each one out loud to yourself. As you read each one take a minute to notice how it makes you feel and write down your feelings under each one. Really get into it by allowing yourself to experience those feelings.

Example: "I'll never lose weight"

Feelings: depressed, hopeless, failure

What did you notice when doing this exercise?

You probably felt depressed, helpless, sad, angry, afraid, lonely or something similar. You might even be feeling a bit down right now.

The point of doing this exercise is to get you to understand the connection between your thoughts, beliefs and outcomes and how this mental stress creates your emotional state which negatively affects your ability to reach your weight loss goals.

If you are constantly thinking and believing these kinds of things and experiencing the negative feelings attached to each thought or belief how in the world do you expect to ever get the body you desire?

That's why you you're not getting the results you want.

Sure you can argue that the reason is because you aren't eating right or exercising enough but the REAL reason why you aren't doing either of these is because of the negative thoughts and beliefs you carry around that are sabotaging you.

That's why you eat *'bad'* foods or skip workouts even though you know you shouldn't.

Take a look at anyone who has vibrant health and a lean, toned attractive body. Do you think they constantly think and believe negatively about their bodies and themselves? Do you think they let a lack of time or motivation stop them from working out?

Not a chance.

Understand that these beliefs do not support you or your goals in any resourceful way and that it's time to let them all go. Don't blame or berate yourself for having these thoughts and beliefs. Just know that there are lessons you were supposed to learn from them and that you have learned those lessons and can now let the negative thoughts and beliefs go.

Now, you're going to let each negative thought or belief go by reframing each one in a positive way. Reframing is simply re-writing each thought or belief in a positive way that supports your goal.

Action Step: Reframe each negative thought or belief into a positive affirmation and write each one down on paper

Example: "I can't lose weight" might become "I am losing weight and on my way to my goal weight of ____lbs"

Make copies and keep your new positive affirmations in a few places where you will see them every day. Examples include: the refrigerator, the bathroom mirror, posted on your computer, on a 3x5 note card (keep in your pocket), on the dashboard of your car.

Read these affirmations out loud at least twice a day every day.

Now, that you've created new beliefs that will serve to support your weight loss goals there's one more critical component you'll need to make it even more powerful.

You're about to discover the secret to developing unstoppable motivation...

Chapter 4
<u>Getting To Know Your 4 'W's:</u>
The Secret To Unstoppable Motivation

If you've ever wondered why you can't seem to find the motivation to stick with your fitness program this will solve the problem once and for all.

It's a simple process I call my 4 W's method and is designed to help you uncover a source of unstoppable motivation that will carry you toward your goal even during the those difficult challenges that will come your way.

Make no mistake the 4 W's process you are about to experience is extremely powerful.

Here's another secret about motivation you may not know...

...You will never find the motivation you need from anything or anyone outside of yourself. All the motivation you're looking for is already within you.

If this sounds a bit crazy to you consider this:

- Looking for something or someone outside of yourself for motivation to get you to your goal will <u>NEVER</u> work because people and things are imperfect and beyond your ability to control which means they are unpredictable and at some point will let you down.

By looking outside of yourself for motivation you give up your power to something or someone else and you become dependent upon that person or thing to achieve your goals. In other words, you allow forces outside of you to control your results. As soon as the very thing you need from the person or thing suddenly changes or is no longer available you will lose your motivation.

- If you are not motivated it isn't because you're lazy...the real reason you're not motivated is because you don't really know why you're doing what you're doing.

- Once you have a <u>BIG</u> enough reason why you'll find all the motivation you need inside of you.

So, let's go through the 4-W's...

W #1: What Do You Really <u>WANT</u>?

I'm going to be blunt here by saying that one of the reasons you haven't achieved long-term weight loss is because quite frankly, you don't know what you want.

Of course you think you know what you want after all you want to lose weight, you want a flat stomach, you want to tone up, you want to increase your energy levels and so on. The problem with having goals like these is that they lack one critical component...

...SPECIFICITY

Here's the deal. Your mind is an extremely powerful tool. It's the very thing we use to get what we want.

For example, if you've ever lost your car keys and needed to drive somewhere you focused your mind like a laser-beam on finding your keys.

It's the same for anything we become determined to do or have. Our mind seeks out information to get what it is that we want. We become so focused that everything else becomes somewhat invisible to us.

But, you have to know exactly what it is that you want because you can't hit a target you're not aiming at.

In other words, you need to know exactly what achieving your goal looks like for you.

Wanting to lose weight is a nice start but let me ask you this...

...In 6 months from now if you got on your scale and only lost 1 pound would you be happy with that result?

After all, you would have achieved your goal of losing weight right?

Obviously, you wouldn't be very thrilled with this result because although you lost weight chances are you had a bigger number in mind.

On the other hand, you may reach a goal you want and never realize it because you haven't established the goal achievement criteria.

For this purpose it's important to know with 100% clarity exactly what you want. Your mind works best with specific details such as numbers and dates.

A specific goal includes important details such as one or more of the following *(or something similar)*:

- ✓ a specific body weight

- ✓ a certain body fat percent

- ✓ a certain clothing size

- ✓ specific measurements

A specific goal also includes an exact date to achieve the goal by (*a deadline*). Without a deadline there is no sense of urgency to achieve your goal. You can drag it on and on without ever achieving it and instead always be *'working on it'*.

If you want to achieve your goal you must have a specific target to aim at. Get out a sheet of paper and write down exactly what it is that you want along with a deadline in which you are going to achieve it.

Example: *"To reach a body weight of (insert goal bodyweight here) lbs by (insert deadline here, include month, date and year)."*

Action Step: Go ahead and write down specifically what you WANT

W #2: WHY Do You Want It?

So now you know what you want. But, that's not enough to stay on track toward achieving your goal until you know your *'why'*. You must know why you want it and your reason must be big enough to keep you focused on getting what it is that you want.

I have had clients in the past who said their goal was to be healthy and they would *'like to lose about 10 lbs'*.

Now, if this is a goal that really excites you and drives you every single day to achieve it then so be it. I'm not here to tell you what your goal should or should not be.

However, these past clients *(along with many other people)* really wanted to lose more along the lines of 20 or even 30+ lbs but in the past they had either tried diets and workout routines that did not produce the outcome they wanted or they weren't prepared to make the sacrifices they needed which often meant getting rid of the deserts, the fast food, the *'just a few'* chips, cookies, candy and other things that were keeping them from achieving their goal.

They wanted to have their cake and eat it too...literally.

But, they did not have a big enough reason driving them to achieve their weight loss goals. Because of this, they weren't willing to take all the necessary steps and accepted that they would not achieve the goal they really wanted and instead set their expectations to a much lower 10 lbs because they felt it was more *'realistic'*.

Again, there's nothing wrong with a 10 lb weight loss goal unless it's not what you really want.

Ironically, most of these clients never even reached the 10 lb goal they set.

Why?

Because even though it may have been more realistic the fact is that deep down it wasn't what they really wanted and as a result, it did not motivate them to stay on course.

Without a big enough reason to achieve your goal you'll NEVER stay motivated long enough to get it.

On the other hand, had these clients looked beyond the weight itself and discovered their *'why'* they could have practically guaranteed their success.

When we want something bad enough we'll do everything in our power to get it.

It really isn't about losing weight but the payoff we get from achieving the goal that drives us to achieve it.

Knowing your want is a great starting point but it's still not enough to keep you on track to reaching your goal. You must know with 100% clarity WHY you want your goal. So, now is the time to sit quietly without any distractions such as radio, television, people, etc and determine this. Only you know the real answer. Without being completely honest you'll only be kidding yourself about achieving your goal. However, once you discover the reason why you want your goal you'll feel a sense of excitement and motivation from within yourself.

You'll need to do some serious soul searching by digging into each answer you come up with and asking yourself *'why is this important to me?'*

Use the following questions or others that you come up with:

- What is it you're looking to get from achieving the goal you want?

  Example: I want to lose 25 lbs so I will look and feel better

- Why is getting it important to you?

Example: Because I used to be in great shape back in college when I played baseball and now I'm so out of shape, I feel horrible and I'm worried about my high blood pressure and cholesterol levels

- What will happen if you do not achieve it?

  Example: My father had high blood pressure and cholesterol and died at an early age. I'm worried that the same thing may happen to me if I don't do something about it. My family needs me and I can't stand the thought of not being there for them

- How will achieving it improve your life?

  Example: I won't have the fear of suffering a heart attack or stroke and not being there for my family. I'll be around to see my kids grow up, to enjoy family vacations and live a long life with my wife

- What specifically will change for you by achieving your goal?

  Example: I'll reach my goal weight of 175lbs, my blood pressure and cholesterol will drop to a healthy level, I won't have to live a life on dangerous medications, I'll have more energy to keep up while playing with my kids and I'll feel more attractive to my wife

The example above may seem a bit extreme and out of the ordinary but this or something similar is actually quite common. However, most of the time we think of a goal we want we tend to stop after the first thought such as in the example above *'I want to lose 25 lbs so I will look and feel better'*.

But, as you can see, the weight itself was not the true source of motivation for this individual.

He had to determine why achieving this goal was important to him. As you can see, his reason for achieving the goal wasn't really about his weight but because he was worried that his present condition might result in the same fate as his father. That's the motivating factor he needs to stay in touch with to keep him on track to achieving his weight loss goal.

Exercise: Now it's your turn. On your sheet of paper:

Action Step: Write down the real reason WHY you want your goal

W #3: WHAT will you need to do to achieve your goal?

Knowing your want and why are important but now you need to have a plan to achieve your goal.

There's a saying that goes *'failing to plan is planning to fail'* and without having a plan of action you stand very little chance of ever achieving your goal.

Your plan begins by knowing what you will need to do to achieve your goal.

On a sheet of paper list everything you can think of that you must do to achieve your goal. Do this to the best of your ability and leave nothing out. You will need to be completely honest here as leaving the things out that you may not want to do or don't particularly like will make it less likely to ever achieve your goal.

Action Step: Write down exactly WHAT you must do to achieve your goal (list everything you can think of)

W #4: Are you WILLING to do what it takes to get it?

This is where you will find out just how serious and committed you are to your goal. You've done a lot of searching so far and now you'll put yourself to the test to determine if you're ready, willing and able to do what it takes to see your goal through to the end.

Let's briefly discuss what each of these means.

- ✓ Ready- You no longer want to *'try'* to lose weight. You realize you MUST lose weight and there is no other alternative.

- ✓ <u>Willing-</u> You accept what it is you need to do and are 100% committed to doing it.

- ✓ <u>Able-</u> You will find the way to do what it takes to achieve your goal no matter what. This is not suggesting doing anything unhealthy but rather you are not interested in why you don't have the time or any other excuses as to why you cannot or will not take all the necessary steps to achieve your goal.

Achieving your goal is going to require consistent action that you and only you can provide. Nothing and no one else can do this for you and therefore, the results you get or do not get are entirely up to you.

If you are not willing to do what it takes then you cannot realistically expect to achieve your goal right?

Take out your *'must do'* list you created during the last exercise as you will be reviewing it now.

Action Step: Go over each item on your 'must do' list and determine if you are 100% ready, WILLING and able to do it by marking a 'Y' for yes or 'N' for no (be completely honest with yourself on this)

Now go over each of your *'Y's* and *'N's* and see how many of each you have. Based on your own answers determine if you are absolutely committed to doing what it takes to achieve the results you want.

For example, if you listed 12 things you must do to achieve your weight loss goals but you determined that you are only willing and able to do 6 of them what are your chances of achieving your goal?

Not very good are they? But, you have a choice.

Your first option is to just accept the fact that although you can achieve your weight loss goal you just aren't ready, willing or able to put forth the effort it takes to get there.

If this is your choice then understand that this outcome is YOUR creation and that you will NEVER reach your weight loss goal but do not complain or make excuses as to why you don't have the body you want.

The other option is to really buckle down with fierce determination to let nothing stand in your way.

There is no room for excuses as to why you cannot or will not do everything it takes to reach your goal as long as it doesn't involve anything dangerous or unhealthy.

It's time to stop arguing for your limitations and really get after it.

If you're ready to give it another go then get out your list and go back over it. Find all of your 'N's' and honestly ask yourself if you are 100% willing and able to turn that 'N' into a *'Y'*. The more *'Y's'* you have the better your chances are of achieving your goal.

If, and only if, you can honestly turn every *'N'* into a *'Y'* you're practically guaranteed to achieve your goal. How could you fail if you are 100% ready, willing and able to do whatever it takes to achieve it?

You can't.

It's simply a matter of finding the right program that works for you.

Fortunately, you have already found it in this book.

All you need now is to be completely committed to taking the actions you listed and implementing the principles in this book until you achieve your goal.

You've accomplished quite a bit so far haven't you?

You've come to realize how negative mental stress leads to negative emotional stress and hormonal changes that sabotage your weight loss efforts.

You've uncovered the negative thoughts and beliefs that have been holding you back from achieving the body you want.

You've learned how to use your negative thoughts and beliefs to get the results you want by reframing them into positive affirmations.

You've also discovered your 4 W's...

...what you *want*...

...*why* you want it...

...*what* you need to do to get it...

...and if you're 100% *willing* and able to do it.

That's probably much more than you expected, right?

Most diet and exercise programs fail to address these critical issues which is why you haven't been able to achieve lasting weight loss. Without the proper mindset even the best diet and exercise program on the planet will be doomed to fail you.

But, by reprogramming your TBAR© Cycle and using the 4 W's process to establish the proper mindset needed to achieve your goals you are practically guaranteed to succeed!

Now, with the proper mindset you're ready to address the next most important piece of the puzzle which is...

Chapter 5

The 'Little-Known' Truth About Nutritional Stress

The Secrets Health & Fitness Experts Aren't Telling You

One of the biggest challenges I've seen over the years in those struggling with their weight is a lack of energy and motivation. Many individuals do not sleep well or enough and wake up feeling exhausted most of the time. They rely on stimulants like caffeine or sugary snacks to get them through their day only to come home from work emotionally, mentally and physically exhausted.

It's no wonder why sticking to an exercise program is difficult for so many. Many people believe this is just how it is when you get *'older'* or that they're simply *'out of shape'*. But, the real reason is often related to poor nutrition.

Poor nutrition can stress out your body every bit as much as physical, mental and emotional stress.

In this chapter we are going to focus on nutritional stress by understanding the effects certain foods (even many so-called *'healthy'* foods) have on you and your ability to lose weight. Once you know what you should be eating and are able to implement that knowledge into your daily lifestyle, exercise becomes a simple addition.

It is also important to understand that no amount of physical activity will offset poor nutritional choices. As the saying goes *"you cannot out train a bad diet"*. You might be thinking that you already know what foods you should be eating and that you're simply just not doing it.

But, if you believe that all you need to do is eat fewer calories, less carbs, watch your fat intake, eat more protein and get 5-6 small meals per day you're about to get a rude awakening. The truth is you don't know what to do.

I'm not saying this to be arrogant or rude but because many of the *'healthy'* eating strategies that most health and fitness experts and even doctors recommend are not only keeping you from losing weight but are wreaking havoc on your energy levels and your health as well.

This may come as a shock to you and you might not believe me. That's alright. All I ask is that for the time being you put aside any disbeliefs. At the end of this chapter if you still don't agree with me you can always take your original beliefs back.

Fair enough?

Good. Let's move on then...

The Truth You Haven't Heard About Diets

If you've tried eating healthy to lose weight before you've probably tried anything from low-carb or no-carb to low-fat or no-fat to low-calorie or very-low calorie to high protein diets or point tracking diet programs without any real long-term success.

You may have lost weight on a diet only to gain it all back with *'interest'* a short time later or you may be stuck at your current weight where no matter what you do nothing is working.

As you will soon see, you haven't failed but rather diets have failed you.

Most diets are focused on strategies like reducing calories, carbohydrates, fat, sugar and other similar tactics. But, the one thing they all fail to account for is stress.

Yes, you read that right.

If you're wondering what stress could possibly have to do with what you eat and how much you weigh you'll be surprised. When we think of stress we often tend to think of the negative things such as coming up with money to pay the bills, completing a work project by a certain deadline, having an argument with loved one or something similar.

But, rarely do we ever consider the effects stress can have on our bodies in relation to the foods we consume. The foods we eat can cause stress that produces digestive problems, muscle and joint pain, depression, constipation, immune system suppression, abnormal blood pressure, poor sleep, insulin resistance, ill health and weight gain.

And, this stress isn't limited to junk foods. The truth is that many of the foods we think of as being healthy for us are producing these and many other problems but most of the time we don't even realize it because we become desensitized to the effects of food over longer periods of time. We feel the way we do so often and have felt this way for so long that it seems normal.

We tell ourselves that the reason we are tired all the time is because we are overweight and out of shape, that our aches and pains are due to *'weak'* knees or a *'bad'* back, our shoulder problems are the result of *'old age'* or that medications are the cure for our health problems. We place blame on just about any and everything other than what we are putting in our mouths. In reality, our weight problems, nagging aches and pains, lack of energy and ill health are all symptoms telling us that something somewhere within our bodies is wrong.

One former client of mine was in her 50's, wanted to lose weight and suffered from chronic muscle and joint pain that limited her ability to play golf which was one of her favorite hobbies. Even though she exercised regularly the pain persisted and her weight wouldn't budge.

At first glance it would have been easy to dismiss this as part of the aging process and tell her to just accept it and that she would need to limit her activity level and perhaps choose a less physically stressful form of activity.

But, I've discovered that regardless of a person's age most can still participate in their favorite activities with the proper diet and exercise program. But, an exercise program without the right diet will get limited results at best.

Most activities and movements are not *'bad'* for us. If you don't believe me look at how toddlers move. They squat down, stand up, bend over, turn and twist, push and pull. But, you never hear of a toddler throwing out their back, rolling an ankle or twisting a knee.

We all performed these movements as toddlers and as kids growing up but somehow we think that just because we've become older we're suddenly unable to perform them?

I don't know about you but I've never heard any voices or read any signs saying *'Now that you're over 40 many of the movements and activities you've been performing are bad for you'.*

It's not the movements and activities that are causing problems. It's a combination of factors resulting from a lack of physical conditioning to perform movements and activities safely and effectively coupled with inadequate nutrition. Over a significant length of time a lack of physical conditioning leads to muscle imbalances where certain muscles become excessively tight or strong while others become excessively loose or weak.

The weaker muscles lose their ability to function properly which leads to compensation strategies during many movements we perform. These compensation strategies overwork the stronger muscles and lead to repetitive stress, pain and/or injuries.

The result of inadequate nutrition can result in a host of problems two of which are weight gain and muscle and joint pain.

Eating the wrong foods can lead to digestive problems, inflammation and muscle and joint pain as undigested food particles make their way into the bloodstream where they can become embedded in nerve, muscle and joint tissues.

After assessing my client I came to the conclusion that her weight and joints were not the actual cause of her problems. They were a symptom that something somewhere in her body was wrong. I came to the conclusion that the primary cause of her weight struggles and physical pain were related to her diet and recommended some significant nutritional changes.

It took her a while to fully commit to the changes I recommended but once she did she made amazing progress. The pain that had plagued her for so long began to disappear. On top of that she lost 35 pounds within 3 months and was able to regularly play 18 holes of golf pain-free.

Dieting to lose weight, taking medications for chronic pain or consuming stimulants like caffeine and sugar to increase your energy levels are all backwards approaches that only address the *symptoms* of the problem while ignoring the *causes*. You come off the diet and the weight comes back. You stop taking medication and the pain returns. The caffeine and sugar wears off and your energy levels plummet. It becomes extremely difficult to lose weight and keep it off when you're only managing the symptoms.

The Biggest Factor That Influences Weight Loss

We have been conditioned to use exercise to burn calories for weight loss. But, given the previous information we know exercise only contributes a small amount to the overall picture.

This brings up an important question...

...Which works best for losing weight diet or exercise?

Exercise is a significant component of any health and fitness program however the biggest factor that influences weight loss is your diet.

"Believe it or not, most research trials examining the weight loss caused by very low calorie diets found that adding exercise did little to increase weight loss beyond what the diet alone could achieve. It was the diets that seemed to do all the work."

"This conclusion has been found over and over again in published research. Donnelly et al. did a second trial that was published in 1993 showing that weight training could increase muscle size while women followed an 800-calorie per day diet, but it could not improve weight loss or fat loss. Similar results have been found by research conducted by Kraemer in 1997, Bryner in 1999, Janssen in 2002 and Wang in 2008 just to name few examples. As you can see, exercising for weight loss has been studied quite extensively and repeatedly proven to be less effective then we have been led to believe."-Pilon, 2010.

While exercise is much needed the role it plays in weight loss is secondary to your diet and influences metabolism primarily by increasing or maintaining muscle and secondly by contributing to energy expenditure.

This is not to suggest that exercise is not important or all that is needed to lose weight and keep it off is a balanced diet.

Dieting without exercise fails to provide the stimulus needed to maintain muscle and mobilize fat stores, water and toxins. Long-term dieting in the absence of exercise leads to stress resulting in muscle loss, a slower metabolism and weight rebound.

It's not a question of one or the other but rather a better understanding of how diet and exercise work together to produce weight loss.

Most health and fitness experts promote exercise to burn calories for weight loss and a diet that contributes to the calorie deficit and supports the exercise program. However, this is a backwards approach. Our diet has the biggest impact on weight loss and body fat reduction and exercise supports our diet not the other way around.

Therefore our diet is the primary component responsible for weight loss and exercise supports our diet in two ways: 1) as a means to keep our metabolic rate high by maintaining or building muscle (2) as a contributing source of energy expenditure to compliment our diet and support weight loss.

The word *'diet'* is associated with eating less. Eating less is typically achieved through calorie reduction by eating less or limiting one or more nutrients.

Reducing calories or limiting nutrients results in a nutrient deficit. Your body requires a certain amount of nutrients that provides the energy to function its' best. The bigger the nutrient deficit becomes the less energy you have available and the more stressful it is on your body. The greater the stress the slower your metabolism becomes and the harder it is to lose weight and keep it off.

The key to maximizing weight loss and body fat reduction is to consume the **maximum** amount of nutrients your body needs to function its' best and your body needs them all; carbohydrates, protein, fat, water, vitamins and minerals.

This is the opposite of how most weight loss diets work. Most diets focus on consuming the minimum amount of food because they are all tied into consuming fewer calories. This is also one of the main reasons most weight loss diets fail over the long-term.

Chapter 6

The Calorie Reduction Controversy
The Truth You Haven't Been Told About Calories

We've been led to believe that losing weight is simply a matter of calories in versus calories out and as long as you burn more calories than you consume or you eat fewer calories than you burn you'll lose weight.

This is known as a *'calorie deficit'*.

If it's true that weight loss is only a matter of calories than everyone would lose weight as long as they remain in a calorie deficit. However, this theory fails to hold up when you look at how many people lose weight by way of a calorie deficit at first and then their weight loss stalls.

They continue to reduce their calories further and may lose a few more pounds but with an increasing level of difficulty. Soon again their weight loss stops and the cat and mouse game of calorie reduction continues. But, there comes a time where weight loss stops no matter how much they reduce their calories or how much they exercise.

According to theory, as long as you remain in a calorie deficit you should continue to lose weight but it just doesn't work this way. So the question is why does calorie reduction stop working after a period of time when it works in so well the beginning?

It's hard to argue that creating a calorie deficit does not work since most people who lose weight do so in this manner. The problem is that while the method does hold some merit, the reason why is misunderstood.

Suppose a person consumes a diet of 2,500 calories per day to maintain his current body weight. This person then decides he wants to lose weight and reduces his calorie intake to 2,000 calories per day creating a calorie deficit of 500 calories per day.

Since 1 pound of fat equals 3,500 calories he should lose 1 pound every week.

At the end of 4 weeks he loses 10 pounds mostly from excess water weight but over the next 4 weeks he only loses 4 pounds and 4 weeks after that he loses only 2 pounds. He figures that his calorie requirements must be lower since he has lost some weight and his current intake no longer puts him in a calorie deficit. So, he figures that reducing his calorie intake by another 500 should do the trick. He is now consuming 1,500 calories per day and manages to lose another 3 pounds over the next 4 weeks but once again his weight loss stops after that.

He notices that he's hungry all the time, feels weak and irritable and doesn't have much energy lately. Since he is having such a difficult time he realizes that he cannot realistically reduce his calories further and decides it's time to start exercising. He exercises moderately 3 days per week for 45 minutes each workout.

After another 4 weeks he only loses 3 pounds and decides he needs to workout longer, more days per week or harder. He exercises vigorously 5 days per week for 60 minutes each workout and after another 4 weeks he loses only 2 pounds. It's as if his body is suddenly fighting against him. Shortly thereafter, he loses his motivation to exercise, has uncontrollable cravings for food and ultimately goes off the diet.

Within a couple of months he gains back all the weight he lost plus a few extra pounds.

This may seem out of the ordinary but I can attest to the fact that although the numbers may vary this is a common scenario for many people. For over a decade I have seen friends, family members and many others struggle with similar situations. On a personal level I too experienced this type of scenario years ago when I struggled with my weight.

So, why does the calorie deficit lose its' effectiveness after the initial period?

Here's the truth...

It's Not The Calories

Every time you reduce the calories you consume you also reduce the amount of nutrients your body receives. Consuming fewer nutrients than your body needs to function its' best creates a 'nutrient deficit'.

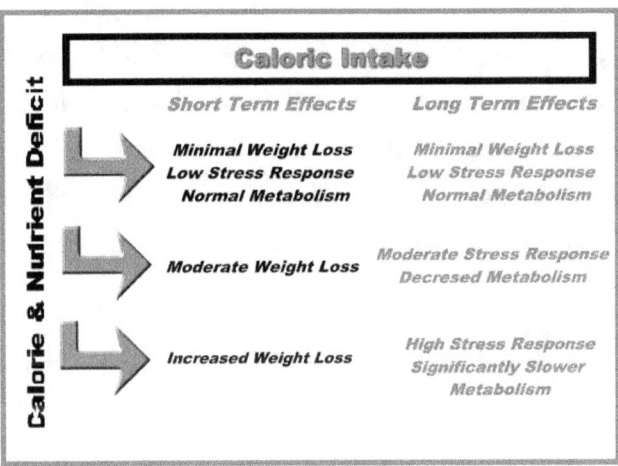

The diagram above represents the short-term and long-term effects associated with varying degrees of a calorie (and nutrient) deficit. The top arrow on the left represents a small deficit. The middle arrow on the left represents a moderate deficit. The bottom arrow on the left represents a large deficit.

A slight calorie deficit creates a slight nutrient deficit but it's often not significant enough for your body to miss and you also do not lose much weight.

A large calorie deficit creates a large nutrient deficit where you lose more weight in the beginning however this also creates a stressful situation to your body because you're using much more energy than you are consuming.

When you create a large nutrient deficit, in order for your body to continue to keep energy expenditure up it has to find a way to produce the energy it's not receiving. Your body does this by using its' own resources. In other words, your body begins feeding off of itself by breaking down its' own tissues.

When you're in a large nutrient deficit for too long your body has a decision to make about which tissues to use. This decision is made by getting rid of the most energy costing tissue and keeping the least energy costing tissue.

The most energy costing tissue in your body muscle. Your muscles are essentially your metabolism. The more muscle you have the more energy you burn and the more efficient your metabolism is. The more efficient your metabolism is the easier it is to lose weight.

But, when you do not have the energy you need and your energy demands exceed what your body is comfortable with this increases your stress level. In an effort to conserve energy your body starts breaking down your own muscle tissue while striving to maintain its' storage of fat. Remember, your muscles are your metabolism so the more muscle you lose the slower your metabolism becomes and the harder it is to lose weight.

Losing Weight By Eating More?

Have you ever known of anyone who struggled to lose weight on a very low calorie diet and then they started eating more and suddenly began losing weight?

So many clients I have worked with over the years went on to lose significant amounts of weight and body fat by eating more rather than eating less.

This goes against everything regarding the calorie deficit theory but it happens. So, how is it possible to lose weight by eating more calories?

It's easy to get confused when you're focused on the calories but it becomes crystal clear when we understand the effects a nutrient deficit has on metabolism. The nutrient deficit created by very low calorie diets is extremely stressful on the body. Under such stress the body fights any and all attempts to lose weight by slowing down energy production.

When calories are increased nutrients are also increased which means the body receives more energy to function so energy production and metabolism begin to speed up.

The point here is that regardless of what all the health and fitness experts are saying it's **not the calories** that are responsible for our weight struggles it's the stress created by the nutrient deficit that's causing the problems.

If you're still not convinced, there are 7 reasons I call the *'7 Flaws Of Calorie Reduction'* that points out why calories are not the problem. This is followed by *'7 Reasons Calorie Counting Does Not Work'*...

7 Flaws Of Calorie Reduction

1. Calories provide our bodies with the nutrients needed to support a healthy metabolism. Reducing calories also reduces the amount of nutrients which **negatively affects metabolism**.
2. The more calories are reduced the bigger the nutrient deficit becomes and the more stress your body experiences. Increased stress leads to elevated cortisol levels that result in muscle breakdown, poor digestion and fat storage making it **more difficult to lose weight**.
3. A significant reduction in calories and nutrients below your body's needs creates a stress response within the body to conserve energy which it does by **slowing down your metabolism**
4. A significant reduction in calories results in a slower metabolism that makes it more difficult to lose weight and **easier to gain weight**

5. **Nutrient deprivation** associated with calorie restriction can lead to: a slower metabolism, weight gain, poor energy levels, decreased mental clarity and focus, hunger, overeating and health problems
6. Most dieters lose weight initially and then reach a point where **weight loss stops** regardless of how much they reduce calories
7. If the only requirement for weight loss is a calorie deficit than weight loss should continue as long as a calorie deficit is achieved; however this is not always the case. In fact, many people lose weight after **increasing their calories**

7 Reasons Calorie Counting Does Not Work

1. Studies show that most individuals **grossly underestimate** how many calories they consume. This means that most people are consuming more calories than they think
2. Studies also show that most people **incorrectly identify portion sizes** resulting in inaccurate calorie tracking
3. Calorie requirements cannot be accurately estimated because your body's **calorie needs can and do change** all the time depending on many factors such as your activity level, hydration status, hormonal environment, and muscle-to-fat ratio. Most of these factors are not possible to measure

without being in a controlled laboratory setting with specialized equipment and testing devices

4. Nutrition charts and food labels only provide **average estimates of calories** making it unlikely to accurately determine how many calories a certain food contains. In other words, if you eat the same meal at your favorite restaurant 5 times it is highly unlikely that you will be consuming the same number of calories each time

5. All calories are **not equal.** We know there are differences between the types of nutrients such as *'good'* and *'bad'* carbs and fats even though the calorie content of each nutrient is the same. All carbohydrates contain 4 calories per gram and all fats contain 9 calories per gram. But, even though the calories are the same results vary depending on the quality of nutrients consumed. If all calories were equal we could eat chips, French fries and soda all the time and get the same results as we would eating fresh vegetables and fruits but we all know it doesn't work this way.

6. The amount of calories you consume may not be the same amount your body actually uses. There are certain **foods that our bodies are not meant to digest** and cannot absorb properly. Foods that contain chemicals, additives or preservatives may not be completely absorbed. Just because you eat

or drink it does not mean your body can actually use it.

7. Nutrient absorption depends on the **quality** of food consumed rather than the **quantity.** Consuming nutritionally deficient, processed and refined or other toxic foods leads to incomplete digestion and digestive problems. These foods can end up stuck like paste along the walls of your intestines for weeks, months and sometimes years and prevent your body from absorbing the nutrients it needs.

The Secret To Controlling Your Weight

If you were to examine your body under the right microscope you would see billions of tiny cells tightly bound together. Your entire body is made up of individual cells. Everything from your muscles, bones, skin, hair, organs; all of it is just cells. Every cell of your body has a specific function which must be maintained in order to have optimal health, vitality and even to lose weight.

In fact, the secret to controlling your weight is providing your cells with the right amount of high-quality nutrients. The function of your body as a whole depends on the health of your cells. Healthy cells require energy in the form of nutrients (carbohydrates, protein, fat, vitamins, minerals and water).

If you don't provide your cells with enough energy they cannot function properly and become compromised. To understand this better think of a time when you were completely exhausted after a long day. You may have wanted nothing more than to get home and relax when you suddenly remembered you have your exercise class and you really want to lose that extra weight. So, you drag yourself to the health club and somehow got through your workout but at much less than 100% effort because you did not have enough energy to do so. Now, had you been completely rested you could have given your all to that workout because you would have had the energy needed to do so.

Well, the same thing happens to all of those cells that produce the hormones that control your metabolism. Give them the energy they need and your metabolism stays high but short change those cells and your metabolism slows down. When your cells become compromised you will have an extremely difficult time losing weight. You also become a magnet for colds, the flu, chronic fatigue, and other types of sickness and disease.

In Other Words:

HEALTHY CELLS = HEALTHY METABOLISM = HEALTHY WEIGHT

UNHEALTHY CELLS = UNHEALTHY METABOLISM = UNHEALTHY WEIGHT

When you give your body the energy it needs you will find that those cravings you get telling you to EAT, EAT, EAT will disappear and you will intuitively know when you've eaten enough. Overeating will become extremely difficult and unlikely which will help regulate your appetite and food intake.

The bottom line is this:

Calories are not the reason you're struggling with your weight.

So, if calories are not the primary reason responsible for our weight problems then what is?

Chapter 7

Food Toxicity: The Untold Story
How 'Healthy' Foods Are Keeping You Fat

Everything we eat affects us and either moves us closer toward our health and weight loss goals or further away from them.

If we eat foods our bodies are not meant to digest we can experience problems such as inflammation, digestive problems, weight gain, immune system suppression, food intolerances and a host of other undesirable conditions.

Unfortunately, these problems are not limited to *'junk'* foods. Many so-called healthy foods cause these problems as well.

The following are 5 *'healthy'* foods that are sabotaging your efforts to lose weight by keeping you fat.

5 'Healthy' Foods That Are Keeping You Fat

1. Reduced calorie, reduced fat, low-carb, low-fat, fat free

These weight loss *'friendly'* foods are low in calories, carbs or fat however they do not satisfy your appetite for very long which often leads to increased hunger and overeating throughout the course of the day. Many of these foods also contain a high amount of sugar which leads to blood sugar imbalances, increased appetite, fat storage and immune system suppression.

2. Multi-grain, whole grain, whole wheat

Consumption of grains poses several potential problems. One problem is phytic acid, a mineral blocker present in the bran of all grains and in the coating of seeds and nuts. Phytic acid neutralizes digestive enzymes, inhibits the absorption of calcium, magnesium, iron, copper and zinc and can lead to digestive problems.

The process of sprouting grains breaks down phytic acid, increases vitamin content and inactivates carcinogens called *'alfatoxins'*. When choosing grains look for organic sprouted grain products.

However, consuming sprouted grains does not account for another problem which is gluten intolerance.

'Many people cannot digest gluten—a protein found in wheat and some other grains that forms the structure of bread dough—and suffer from a mild to severe gluten intolerance. Possible symptoms of gluten intolerance include: abdominal pain and cramping, bloating and flatulence, bone and joint pain, chronic diarrhea, emotional disturbances such as anxiety and depression, fatigue (especially after eating gluten-containing foods), infertility, painful skin rash, hormone disruption, irritable bowel syndrome (IBS) and celiac disease, weight gain or the inability to lose weight.'-De Los Rios, 2009.

Many minerals are reduced in processed white and wheat flour compared to whole grains leaving them nutritionally deficient. For over 50 years conventionally farmed American grains have been low in protein content and quality.

'The US tried giving its surplus grains to countries with starving populations, but they would not accept grains from the US if grains from any other countries were offered. This was because the deficient US grains did little to maintain or improve the health of the starving.'-Chek, 2004.

3. <u>Pre-packaged and frozen foods</u>

Many of these are cleverly marketed as healthy due to their low calorie, carbohydrate or fat content. The truth is that these foods are processed leaving them nutritionally deficient. They also contain additives and preservatives that your body is not meant to digest. So, the minimal nutrition in these foods may not actually be absorbed by your body.

4. **Conventional dairy**

Contrary to popular belief, milk does not do a body good due to the processes of pasteurization and homogenization.

Pasteurization is the process of heating the milk to kill off bacteria. This process not only destroys unhealthy bacteria; it also destroys healthy bacteria leading to lactose intolerance in some individuals. This heating process also damages or destroys the milk's vitamins and proteins. Pasteurized dairy can also cause serious illness when it has gone bad.

Homogenization is the process of passing milk through a fine filter to decrease the size of the fat molecules. The fat molecules become evenly dispersed so there is no visible separation of the cream from the milk. This not only affects the absorption of fats needed by the body but it can also negatively affect protein absorption because proteins that are typically digested may not be broken down properly which increases the chance of incomplete digestion. Some of these undigested proteins can make their way into the bloodstream causing inflammation and activating the immune system leading to allergic reactions and intolerance.

- *Calcium-* It has been suggested that <u>50% of the calcium in dairy products is unusable</u> by the body.

- *Growth Hormone-* Cows are commonly injected with rBGH which stimulates milk production and overstresses the cows. It has been reported that cows injected with rBGH are <u>80% more susceptible to infection</u> for which they must be given antibiotics to treat. Unfortunately, the hormones and antibiotics given to the cows end up in the milk supply as well.

- *Yogurt-* On a positive note, yogurts containing microorganisms are very beneficial to the digestive system. These *'friendly'* bacteria are necessary for the production of several vitamins. Acidophilius and bifidus also increase the bioavailability of calcium, iron and other minerals. Those who are lactose intolerant can often tolerate quality yogurt.

5. **Caffeine (and other stimulants)**

Caffeine is an irritant and stimulates the sympathetic nervous system (SNS). The SNS is your body's response to stress.

SNS Stimulation→Increased Cortisol→Liver Releases Glycogen→Increased Blood Glucose (blood sugar) Levels→Increased Insulin→Fat Storage

Caffeine stays active in the body for about 6 hours and also causes peristalsis (involuntary rhythmic contractions in the digestive tract) to eliminate it. The problem here is that foods consumed at or around the time of caffeine ingestion may not be properly digested and absorbed.

Caffeine also creates an acidic environment that the body must use its' own resources to neutralize. These resources are taken in the form of calcium from your bones and protein from your own muscle tissue!

Frequent caffeine consumption can also lead to adrenal fatigue and adversely affect the PNS which is your body's stress recovery system.

'In addition, caffeine:

- *Affects your ability to absorb and use folate, vitamin B12 and vitamin B6*
- *Is linked to raised cholesterol*
- *Negatively affects insulin levels*
- *Contributes to rheumatoid arthritis*
- *Increases the risk of heart disease*
- *Increases the risk of stroke'*

   -Moy, 2010.

More On Food Toxicity

Most weight loss diets are focused on calorie reduction by consuming fewer calories overall or restricting one or more nutrients (ex: low-carbohydrate diets). However, calorie and nutrient restriction fails to account for the most important factor; the effects all foods and drinks we consume have on the body.

For example, many low calorie and low fat foods are toxic and stressful to the body resulting in the storage of fat, water and toxins. A perfect example of this is the number of people who consume diet sodas containing ZERO calories yet struggle to lose weight. Again, it's not the calories that are responsible it's the toxic overload from the chemicals and additives.

Our bodies are not designed to digest these and other foreign substances and when they enter the body they are transported to the liver for detoxification. However, the liver can only handle so much at once and if we keep ingesting toxic foods and substances, regardless of their calorie content, they are stored inside our fat cells along with water to help dilute the toxins.

Toxic foods overload the liver and activate a defense mechanism where the body tries to remove them from the bloodstream in order to prevent the toxins from causing stress and damage to your body. One of the liver's many functions is detoxification but when overloaded it cannot perform this efficiently.

These toxins (along with excess water) are stored in your fat cells until your liver can deal with them.   And, when your liver is overburdened with toxins anything you consume sits in your digestive tract until your liver is ready to deal with it.

The problem here is that during this time your body is not receiving enough of the nutrients it needs and before long your brain starts sending you signals to eat again. And, when you eat you pile more food on top of the food that's still waiting to be digested.

It's similar to when a sink drain gets clogged up. If you keep pouring water down the drain it just backs up. That's what happens inside our bodies. We become *'clogged'* up and our bodies end up storing much of the food as fat regardless of how many calories we consume.

Most diets are focused on short-term outcomes that provide a temporary *'quick-fix'* but rarely do the results last. Many of these leave dieters in worse health than when they began because they fail to address food toxicity.

Controlling calorie intake alone is not an effective long-term solution.

Once toxins stop entering the body, the liver can do its' job. Stored toxins are then released and subsequently eliminated (along with excess water).

Therefore, by eliminating or significantly reducing toxins you experience results such as: weight loss, body fat reduction, decreased muscle and joint pain, increased energy and vibrant health.

Since calorie reduction strategies are flawed, you will be relieved to know that you do not need to count calories, track points, weigh or measure foods, eliminate carbs or fat to lose weight, reduce body fat and improve your health.

Instead, you will lose weight and stubborn fat quickly while improving your energy levels and overall health by following the 14 P's of stress free nutrition covered in the next chapter.

But, first let's look at another important piece of the weight loss puzzle...

Chapter 8

Determining Your Metabolic Profile

How To Unleash The Power Of Your Metabolism

Most diets use a 'one-size-fits-all' approach to losing weight by attempting to blame everyone's weight problems on one thing. A great example is low-carbohydrate diets.

Have you ever wondered why some people get great results on a low-carb diet while others feel lousy and fail to get results?

Have you ever noticed how many diet books and programs there are on the shelves of most book stores? With all of these *'solutions'* on the market how do you know which one really works?

The simple answer is all of them work...at least to some degree.

But, not all of these approaches work for everyone and the ones that do often only work for a short time.

The reason why a particular approach works for some but not for others is due in large part to our metabolic profile or type. The book '*The Metabolic Typing Diet'* documents the studies of various populations of tribes that were not exposed to the refined and processed foods containing sugar and hydrogenated oils that exist in today's diet. Instead, they lived on organic, whole foods and animal products that were available depending on where they lived. Their diets were also much higher in vitamins and minerals than the typical American diet of today.

Tribes such as the Eskimos consumed diets that were very high in protein and fat and low in carbohydrates while others such as the Quetchus Indians consumed diets high in carbohydrates and little protein and fat. The common theme among the different tribes was the lack of obesity and disease prevalent in our modern culture.

In fact, as soon as these tribes were exposed to foods and dietary customs of modern civilization they developed the same health problems as industrialized societies.

It all comes down to understanding your unique nutritional needs based what your metabolism is best designed for. Each of us possesses our own specific nutrient requirements based on our genetic make-up. In other words, what works for one doesn't necessarily work for another.

There are 3 metabolic profiles: protein types, carb types, mixed types. The descriptions and guidelines that follow are approximations only. For more information please refer to *'The Metabolic Typing Diet'* by William L. Wolcott and *'How To Eat, Move and Be Healthy'* by Paul Chek.

Protein Types

Protein types metabolize carbohydrates quickly and need more protein and fat to slow the digestion of carbohydrates. Protein types may sleep better and feel rested upon waking if they eat a meal that is higher in fat and protein closer to bedtime (within 2-3 hrs or even less).

Protein types do better on full-fat dairy products. If they eat low-fat yogurts and cheeses, for example, they're usually hungry again in no time.

You are likely a protein type if you:
- Live to eat
- Are still hungry after a high carbohydrate meal
- Sleep well on a full stomach (especially a fatty meal)
- Feel your best after a hearty breakfast
- Prefer fatty, salty foods rather than sweets

Protein type guidelines-Each meal or snack should consist of approximately:

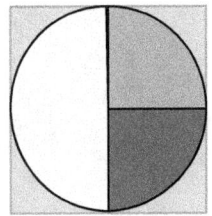
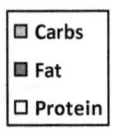

- ☐ Carbs
- ☐ Fat
- ☐ Protein

- ✓ **50% protein**
- ✓ **25% fat**
- ✓ **25% carbohydrates**

Carb Types

Carb types are the opposite of protein types. Carb types do not metabolize fats and proteins as efficiently as protein types and require a proportionately larger amount of carbohydrates. However, this is not a license to eat all kinds of junk foods like chips, cookies, sodas and the like. Regardless of your metabolic profile, carbohydrate sources must consist of real, nutritious food, not junk food even if you feel good after consuming them.

Carb types typically do not feel well eating full-fat dairy products or fatty meats. These foods often make them feel sleepy, lethargic and have cravings for sweets or coffee to increase their energy levels. Carb types feel best consuming light meats like chicken breast, lean meats and light fish.

You are likely a carb type if you:

- Eat to live
- Feel full but hungry after a meal high in protein or fat
- Do not sleep well on a full stomach
- Feel your best after a light breakfast
- Prefer sweets rather than fatty, salty foods

<u>Carb type guidelines</u>-Each meal or snack should consist of approximately:

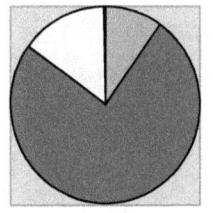

| ▫ Fat |
| ▪ Carbs |
| ▫ Protein |

✓ **75% carbohydrates**

✓ **15% protein**

✓ **10% fat**

Mixed types

Mixed types are a blend of both carb and protein types and go back and forth between the two. This back and forth fluctuation can occur from meal to meal or month to month depending on many different factors. Mixed types must develop keen intuition to understand their bodies' needs at any particular time.

Mixed types will eat like a protein or a carb type most of the time but typically will not feel their best if they stick to one type of diet for too long.

You are likely a mixed type if you:

- Possess most of the characteristics of each profile type
- Go back and forth between the two types
- Feel best when you do not stick with either type of eating for too long

Mixed type guidelines-Each meal or snack should consist of approximately:

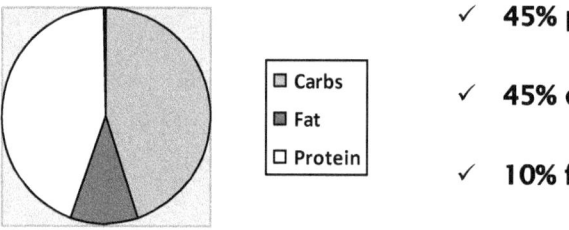

✓ **45% protein**

✓ **45% carbohydrate**

✓ **10% fat**

How Many Meals You Really Need To Lose Weight

For some, eating smaller meals frequently throughout the day is easier on the digestive system and feels best. However, others may feel their best consuming only 2 or 3 meals per day.

While most of the clients I have worked with lost weight eating more food not all of them consumed their food over the 5 or 6 small meals a day often recommended by most health and fitness experts.

Some ate only 3 meals per day and experienced weight loss, reduced body fat and increased energy.

Contrary to what most health and fitness experts say, there is no metabolism boosting magic from eating smaller, more frequent meals nor will you lose muscle or slow down your metabolism by going more than a few hours without food.

It all comes down to your hormones; particularly insulin.

Insulin is a hormone your body releases to store nutrients in your muscle cells, fat cells, liver and other tissues. Glucagon is a hormone your body produces that releases fatty acids from your fat cells. These two hormones are like yin and yang in that when one increases the other decreases. So, when insulin levels increase, glucagon levels and your ability to burn fat decreases.

Insulin levels remain elevated for approximately 2-3 hours following most meals.

The idea of eating smaller meals more frequently throughout the day is thought to keep insulin levels balanced. But, if you consume the same amount of food per day it doesn't really matter if you consume it over the course of 2 meals or 10 meals per day.

Every time you consume food your insulin levels increase so eating more times throughout the day may cause your insulin levels to increase to a lesser degree but the increases happen more often.

Eating bigger meals less often throughout the day may cause more dramatic increases in your insulin levels but they occur with less frequency.

As you can see, there's no right or wrong when it comes to how many times you eat over the course of any given day because there's no *significant* difference between eating smaller meals more often or bigger meals less often. It's more a matter of what works best for you.

Insulin has been shown to increase more dramatically following the consumption of carbohydrates versus protein or fats. Eating a meal containing protein or fat blunts the degree to which insulin levels rise.

So, the degree to which insulin levels rise depends more on *what* you eat rather than how *often* you eat therefore, eating more frequently does not have a significant advantage over eating less frequently.

The 'Starvation Mode' Myth

Most health and fitness experts recommend eating smaller, more frequent meals to avoid the dreaded *'starvation mode'* which is the point at which the body begins using its' own lean tissue to produce energy causing a slowing down of the metabolism and weight gain.

However, the book *'Eat Stop Eat'* documents studies on short-term fasting for periods of 24-72 hours that have shown *increases* in the breakdown and use of fat for energy, growth hormone levels, glucagon (fat releasing) and *decreases* in blood sugar and insulin levels <u>without losing muscle</u>.

Starvation mode is not based on time, it is based on when your body turns to using its' own lean body mass for energy production and based on the research this does not happen for periods lasting longer than 72 hours in the absence of food. Therefore the *'starvation mode'*, muscle loss and metabolic slow down you often hear about cannot occur by eating only 2-3 meals per day.

However, if you over eat on a regular basis or consume a diet that is nutritionally deficient for a significant length of time you will lose muscle, your metabolism will slow down and you will find it difficult to lose weight.

In my experience, the #1 problem with weight gain in people eating 3 or fewer meals per day has little to do with the number of meals they consume and a lot to do with the amount and type of foods they consume.

A diet containing significant amounts of sugar in the form of simple carbohydrates, processed foods, additives and preservatives will lead to uncontrollable food cravings, over eating and weight gain.

The ideal number of meals and snacks per day is the amount that allows you to maintain sufficient energy levels between meals, good mental clarity and focus, a state of well being and the ability to effectively deal with stress.

Nutrient Facts & Sources

Carbohydrates

Carbohydrates are our primary preferred source of energy during physical activity. Our capacity to store carbohydrates is limited and consuming more carbohydrates than you need will result in fat storage. However, not everyone needs a low-carbohydrate diet. We all need a certain amount of carbohydrates that varies from person to person and is determined by our metabolic profile.

Optimum carbohydrate sources include: organic vegetables and fruits, sprouted grain breads*, brown or wild rice*, beans, plain yogurt with active cultures***(no fruit added as they are highly processed and filled with sugar), milk**

*also gluten-free if you are gluten intolerant

**best source is non-pasteurized, non-homogenized, free of hormones and antibiotics

***these are healthy bacteria that support digestion and are usually found near the ingredient label. Look for active cultures such as bifidum and acidophilus

Carbohydrate Guidelines

- Choose organic fruits and vegetables whenever possible

- Even though the sugar in fruits is metabolized more efficiently than refined sugar it is important not to consume too much fruit

- Avoid as many processed carbohydrates as possible including: pastas, breads, cereals and all frozen foods

- If you are gluten intolerant avoid all wheat products including whole wheat, whole grain, multi-grain, soy and teriyaki sauces and lunch meats (most contain gluten)

- Avoid so-called *'healthy'* carbohydrates snacks such as pretzels, crackers, low-fat and low-calorie chips, cookies and similar products as they are highly processed, nutritionally deficient, toxic to the body, often lead to over eating and weight gain

Protein

Protein provides our bodies with the building blocks for repairing body tissues, building and maintaining muscle and is also a source of energy. Protein also helps control appetite by making you feel fuller longer and slows the release of insulin which supports weight loss and body fat reduction.

Protein uses more energy to break down and digest and up to 30% of the calories in protein are used in the process of digestion alone!

Although everyone needs protein not everyone should follow a high protein diet. Consuming more protein than your body can use often results in converting excess protein to fat.

It is important to consume an adequate amount of carbohydrates in your diet because when carbohydrate needs are not met for a significant length of time the body uses protein by breaking down muscle tissue to supply energy which slows down your metabolism.

Most individuals only need between 90-120 grams of protein per day which is easily obtainable by diet alone and therefore supplementation is usually not needed. It is best to consume protein from whole, natural food sources because the protein (and other nutrients) found in most powders and bars undergo processing which makes them unusable by the body.

Conventionally raised cattle and poultry are fed unhealthy grains and given drugs which places undue stress on their bodies. They often become sick and are given antibiotics. The drugs and antibiotics given to these animals make their way into the meats and poultry you eat.

Optimum protein sources include: organic, grass-fed meats, organic, vegetarian-fed poultry, wild seafood, dairy*, beans, raw unroasted nuts

*best source is non-pasteurized, non-homogenized, free of hormones and antibiotics

Avoid fish, seafood and meats that are frozen, farmed, processed, cured or canned as they typically contain additives such as nitrates and nitrites which are used to enhance color and taste but may be carcinogenic (cancer causing).

Protein Guidelines

- Consume protein (and fats) with every meal and/or snack

- Protein and fats help blunt the insulin response and regulates blood sugar levels

- The best protein options are from organic, fresh, natural sources

- Look for fish that are *'wild'* rather than *'farmed'*. Many stores now list this on the price labels in the seafood department

- Fresh vs frozen: Many frozen varieties contain chemicals, additives and preservatives. It is better to purchase fresh and freeze it yourself if needed

- Most protein supplements (powders, bars, etc) are processed which makes the nutrients unusable by the body. It is best to stick with whole, fresh food protein sources
- Buy fresh rather than frozen. Additives, preservatives and chemicals are added to many frozen foods. You can always freeze fresh protein sources if needed

Fats

Fats are essential for optimum health. They provide the building blocks for our cells and for important hormones. There are 2 main categories of fats: saturated and unsaturated.

Saturated fats include foods such as: animal products (fatty cuts of red meat, dark poultry meat), dairy, coconut and palm oil. Saturated fats have been promoted as unhealthy by most health and fitness experts and doctors.

However, here are some facts to consider. There are populations of tribes in areas of the world such as Eskimos who consume diets high in fat and large quantities of meat and live with excellent immunity and cardiovascular health.

There are Swiss people living in isolated mountain villages who eat large amounts of high-fat cheese, cream and raw goats milk yet they are very healthy.

"If, as we have been told, heart disease results from the consumption of saturated fats, one would expect to find a corresponding increase in animal fat in the American diet over the same amount of time as the increase in heart disease. Actually, the converse is true. During the sixty-year period from 1910–1970, the proportion of traditional animal fat in the American diet declined from 83 percent

to 62 percent, and butter consumption plummeted from eight kilograms per person each year to about two. During the past eighty years, the consumption of dietary cholesterol intake has increased only one percent. If saturated fat consumption actually decreased, then what increased? During the same period, the average intake of dietary vegetable oils (in the form of margarine, shortening, and refined oils) increased by about 400%, and the consumption of sugar and processed foods increased by about 60%"- Enig and Fallon. 1999.

Saturated fats have many beneficial functions such as helping protect the liver from toxins, enhancing the immune system and providing stability for strong cell membranes. The saturated fats found in coconut oil, palm kernel oil and organic butter are used primarily for energy production and less likely to be stored as fat. Saturated fats are best used when cooking at high heat temperatures because they are more stable and do not go rancid like unsaturated fats do.

Unsaturated fats include foods such as: avocados, olive oil, flaxseed oil, fish oil, fish, nuts such as almonds, cashews, walnuts, seeds, natural peanut butter, almond and nut butters. Unsaturated fats contain essential fatty acids.

Essential fatty acids (EFA's) are fats that our bodies require but cannot make on their own. These fats must be supplied by the diet. EFA's can be divided into 2 categories: omega 3 and omega 6. The average American diet is high in omega 6 fats so the most important focus in on getting enough omega 3 fats. Omega 3 fats are necessary for the health and development of the brain and nervous system.

Hydrogenated fats (a.k.a. trans-fats or TFA's) are the most dangerous to your health and efforts to lose weight and should be avoided at all costs. TFA's are linked to heart disease, elevated LDL levels (bad cholesterol) and other undesirable health consequences.

Cooking With Fats

Fats should never be heated to the point where they begin to smoke or become discolored because the fatty acids decompose and become damaged.

The best fats for cooking are: organic coconut oil and organic butters. Because of their high fat content they stay stable up to 375 degrees.

Oils that are low in saturated fat and high in monounsaturated fat like olive oil are best when used raw (on salads, etc) or for light sautéing.

Although coconut oil and organic butters are high in fat it's important to remember that saturated fat from organic sources is NOT the cause of weight gain and health problems. Consumption of hydrogenated trans fats are the culprit.

In fact, the saturated fats like those found in organic coconut oil and organic butters are used to help boost the immune system, provide cell membrane structure, calcium absorption in bone, protect the liver from toxins and utilize essential fatty acids.

There is a reason why our bodies produce saturated fats and not essential fats.

Fat Guidelines:

- Consume most of your fat intake in the form of EFA's but also include some saturated fats as well

- Try to avoid hydrogenated fats as much as possible. Look for ingredients that say "hydrogenated" or "partially hydrogenated". You may find these in foods like pretzels, crackers, low-fat and fat-free snacks

- Avoid margarine or shortening and choose organic butter instead. Most stores carry organic butters at affordable prices

- Look out for food labels that contain trans-fats

- Choose snack options such as fresh fruits, raw nuts, natural peanut, cashew, macadamia or almond butter, live yogurts and fresh veggies

- When choosing nut butters the label should list only one kind of nut and salt

- Consume raw nuts that are not roasted as roasting makes the fats rancid

- When eating eggs consume the whole egg as the yolks contain more than 90% of the calcium, iron, phosphorus, zinc, thiamin, B6, folate, and B12, and panthothenic acid of the egg. In addition, the yolks contain ALL of the essential fatty acids. Also, the protein of whole eggs have a better balance of amino acids making whole eggs a better source of protein than egg whites

- The best choice for eggs is vegetarian fed, no hormones or antibiotics given

Our Most Important Nutrient For Weight Loss

The most important nutrient for weight loss is the one that makes up about 70% of our bodies. It's water. Water enables all sorts of processes in our bodies to occur. Unfortunately, most people do not consume nearly enough water. Inadequate water consumption leads to dehydration. Dehydration can lead to hunger, over eating, difficulty losing weight, weight gain, poor performance, cramping, constipation and even back pain.

The problem is that you rarely notice that you are dehydrated until you're thirsty. Most people who rely on thirst as an indicator to drink only put back about 50%-75% of the water they lose and remain in a constant state of dehydration. If you are thirsty you are most likely already dehydrated.

When You're Hungry You're Not Really Hungry

Do you often feel hungry shortly after you've eaten a meal? If so, you aren't really hungry at all. In fact, most of the time we feel hungry is not due to an actual need for food. The chances are that most of us have never actually experienced true hunger.

Of course we need to eat but most of the time we feel hungry we are really thirsty. Our need for water often disguises itself as hunger resulting in over eating and weight gain. This is especially true if you feel hungry soon after you've eaten a meal, first thing in the morning, after a cup of coffee or following a workout. When this happens try drinking 2 cups of water immediately. If your hunger symptoms disappear within a couple of minutes you are likely dehydrated.

How Much Water Do You Really Need?

Most people have no idea how much water they lose during the day nor how much they need. Do your best to consume ½ of your bodyweight in ounces of water per day.

Example: Person weighing 170 lbs

170 / 2 = 85 ounces of water

85 / 8 ounces per cup = approximately 11 cups per day

You will need even more than this if you are physically active or if you consume caffeine. This may seem like too much and you might be thinking that you cannot possibly drink that much water. Remember, our bodies are made up mostly of water. Water is our most important nutrient. In fact, the human body can survive 30 days without food but only 4 to 10 days without water.

Our bodies use water for many different chemical reactions to occur and we lose significant amounts of water every day. Your body cannot produce anywhere near the amount of water it needs nor can it effectively store it.

Most people only put back 50%-75% of the water they lose and remain in a constant state of dehydration.

Another thing to keep in mind is water quality. Most of our water supply is polluted and lacks an adequate amount of minerals our bodies need. Artesian waters contain higher amounts of dissolved solids and are a quality source of water.

If you find that you are urinating frequently upon increasing your water intake this is not a sign of your body *'cleansing'* itself. It means that you're not absorbing enough of the water you're putting in. It's simply going in one end and out the other. Try adding a tiny pinch of unprocessed, unrefined sea salt to your water. This will help your body absorb the water more effectively. You should not actually taste the salt.

Helpful hints for optimal hydration

1. Consume 2 cups of water first thing in the morning

2. Consume 2 cups of water every 1-2 hours depending on your daily needs

3. Weigh yourself before and after exercise and drink 2 cups of water every 30 minutes during exercise

4. Consume 2 cups of water for each pound of body weight lost during exercise.

5. Do not rely on thirst. If you are thirsty you are most likely already dehydrated.

We've uncovered quite a bit of information over the last several chapters haven't we? You understand that diets and calorie reduction strategies are flawed and the negative effects a large nutrient deficit and many so-called *'healthy'* foods can have on your metabolism, your weight and your health.

You've come to realize the importance of eating according to your metabolic profile, how many meals you really need to lose weight and the importance of water. In the next chapter you will discover more foods are the true cause of nutritional stress and weight gain along with the 14 P's that will serve as your guideline to stress free nutrition and the body you want.

Chapter 9

The Principles Of Stress Free Nutrition
The 14 'P's Of Eating For Weight Loss

Most weight loss diets are based on the model of calories in versus calories out.

As you have discovered, calorie reduction is a flawed method and rarely, if ever, do we ever consider the effect that stress can have on our bodies in relation to the foods we consume.

The foods we eat can cause stress that produces digestive problems, muscle and joint pain, depression, constipation, immune system suppression, abnormal blood pressure, poor sleep, insulin resistance, ill health and weight gain.

And, this stress isn't limited to junk foods. The truth is that many of the foods we think of as being healthy for us are producing these and many other problems but most of the time we don't even realize it because we become desensitized to the ill effects of food over longer periods of time. We feel the way we do so often and have felt this way for so long that it seems normal.

You have already learned quite a bit about nutritional stress in the previous chapters but you still might be wondering what you should eat.

There is no easy answer to this question as we all have our own preferences.

However, the key to losing weight, reducing body fat and improving your health starts with nutrition. After all, you could exercise all you want but it's not enough to offset the effects of poor nutrition.

Nutrition comes down to using simple, effective principles rather than ineffective, short-term strategies like counting calories, restricting nutrients like carbohydrates and fat, weighing and measuring foods or tracking points.

It's as simple as reducing as much toxicity from your diet as possible. In the following lists you will come to know the 10 P's to avoid and the 4 P's to include in your diet.

The more of the 10 P's you can eliminate from the first list the better you will look and feel.

Some will come as no surprise to you while other foods in the 10 P's list are those you have been led to believe are healthy. Unfortunately, these foods are anything but and you're probably consuming many of them regularly.

The second list is the 4 P's that should make up the majority of your diet. Include these 4 P's as much as possible and you'll lose those unwanted pounds and inches faster than you can believe while your energy levels and health skyrocket.

Without further ado allow me to introduce the 14 P's of stress free nutrition...

The 10 P's To Avoid:

1. Processed- Avoid lunch meats, cookies, pastas, cakes, pies, breads, products that are canned, bottled, bagged, frozen and ingredients you cannot pronounce

2. Packaged- Foods that come in bags, boxes, ready-made foods, deli counter food, microwavable entrees, frozen foods

3. Powdered- Avoid most nutritional supplements, sauce mixes, seasoning mixes and powdered foods

4. Psuedo-Substances, chemicals, additives and preservatives. Typically used in artificial sweeteners, nutrition bars, conventional regular and decaffeinated coffees (*chemicals are used on the crops and in the decaffeination process*). Choose organic coffees and swiss water processed decaf varieties as these are not treated with chemicals.

5. Pills- Synthetic supplements cannot be used by the body and should be avoided. If using supplements choose whole food varieties

6. Pesticides- Conventional fruits and veggies, coffee beans and soils

7. Phytates- Phytic acid is a mineral blocker found in most grains (*whole grain, whole wheat, multi-grain*). Also most individuals are intolerant to the gluten found in wheat and most grains. Those who

are gluten intolerant should choose organic sprouted grain products

8. <u>Poison</u>- Alcohol is treated as toxic once ingested as in 'in-**toxic**-ated' meaning poison

9. <u>Pasteurized</u>- Conventional dairy products are heavily processed by way of pasteurization that kills off healthy bacteria needed for proper digestion and homogenization that changes the structure of the fats to the point where they cannot be properly absorbed in the body.

10. <u>Physiological stimulants</u>- Those that provide '*false*' energy by stimulating the nervous system such as sugar, caffeine, energy drinks, pills, etc

The 4 P's To Include:

1. Pure- Fresh, whole foods in their natural state such as raw nuts, fruits and veggies

2. Produce- Fresh, organic produce is free of pesticides and chemicals. If organic is not possible all the time then try to limit conventional produce to those items you do not eat the outside or skin (bananas, watermelon, oranges, cantaloupe, etc)

3. Probiotics- Microorganisms that are present in the digestive tract and promote digestion and health. Organic plain yogurts, organic butters

4. Protein- Those free of hormones and antibiotics and not grain fed. If these are not available then buy only fresh meats, poultry and fish instead of frozen.

Include the following protein sources:

- *Poultry- Organic, vegetarian fed, cage free*

- *Red meat- Organic, grass-fed is best*

- *Eggs- Organic, vegetarian fed, cage free*

- *Fish- Fresh, wild not farmed*

Chapter 10

<u>Is Exercise Stopping You From Losing Weight?</u>
Inside Secrets Reveal How Physical Stress Is Really Affecting Your Weight

In this day and age where most people have a gym membership exercise is a way of life. Exercise is necessary for optimal health and weight loss.

Exercise is a form of physical stress that is healthy and beneficial.

But, can physical stress from exercise actually prevent you from losing weight?

The short answer is yes.

We all know the types of individuals who rarely, if ever, exercise, eat too much junk food and complain about their inability to lose weight. I think just about everybody would agree these individuals would benefit from more physical stress in the form of exercise.

But, these aren't the only ones experiencing problems with their weight.

There are also those who eat healthy and exercise regularly yet find themselves dealing with nagging aches and pains or stuck at a point where they cannot reach their weight loss goals no matter how much they exercise or how clean their diet is.

To better understand why this happens we need to take a quick look at what really happens inside our bodies.

The Miracle Of Movement

Our very own lives depend on movement. Movement is how oxygen and nutrients are transported throughout our bodies. Our organs and tissues need a constant supply of oxygen and nutrients to perform their functions and keep us alive.

Even weight loss depends on movement. Losing weight and keeping it off requires exercise. Exercise is dependent upon movement. Therefore, weight loss is the result of movement.

Movement is the result of muscular contraction. Every time our muscles contract a *'pump-like'* effect is created that distributes blood, oxygen and nutrients throughout the body.

Our heart is the center of it all and functions as the delivery system by circulating freshly oxygenated blood throughout our bodies with each powerful beat. This process is repeated an average of 70-75 times per minute 24 hours a day.

Our bloodstream serves as the vehicle that transports oxygen and nutrients to our vital organs, muscles and bodily tissues.

Our muscles do the dirty work by extracting oxygen and nutrients from the bloodstream and pushing out waste and harmful by-products for elimination.

This complex yet elegant relationship operates beyond our awareness.

Movement requires muscular work which helps maintain an efficient metabolism and a strong body. Failure to perform muscular work on a regular basis inhibits movement resulting in decreased energy production, chronic fatigue, muscle breakdown, decreased bone density, weight gain, injuries and health problems.

Lack of movement is associated with increased levels of blood glucose, triglycerides (fatty acids in the blood), cholesterol, insulin, weight gain, fat storage and other undesirable health consequences.

When we consume food the body responds by releasing the hormone insulin. Insulin transports blood glucose to your muscle, liver and fat cells in an effort to reduce blood glucose levels. Glucose is stored in our muscles and liver as glycogen. However, our muscles and liver have a limited storage capacity for glycogen and once full-capacity is reached the remaining blood glucose is stored as fat.

Elevated blood glucose and insulin levels promote weight gain and fat storage.

Muscular work relies primarily on the use of glucose which reduces the amount in the muscles and bloodstream. Lower levels of blood glucose keeps insulin levels balanced and increases the availability of fatty acids for use by the muscles. In other words, lower blood glucose levels can aid weight loss and body fat reduction.

Movement also helps maintain a healthy, efficient digestive system by increasing the rate of nutrient absorption and the removal of waste. Lack of movement can inhibit digestion as food and waste build up along the digestive tract that decreases the ability to absorb nutrients into the bloodstream. This leads to problems including weight gain, constipation, food intolerances, allergic reactions, inflammation and other health problems.

You've Been Secretly Brainwashed

Since movement requires muscular work and weight loss is dependent upon movement this obviously means that in order to lose weight and keep it off exercise is needed.

When it comes to exercise for weight loss most health and fitness experts and doctors recommend the same advice...'eat less and move more' or 'burn more calories than you consume'.

This is based on the first law of thermodynamics that suggests energy cannot be created nor destroyed only transformed or transferred and therefore taking in less energy than your body expends creates an energy deficit the body must compensate for by using energy from its' own storage supply resulting in weight loss.

We measure this energy in units called *'calories'*.

Controlling calories has become a way of life for those seeking leaner bodies and better health through weight loss.

Television infomercials advertise the newest breakthrough cardiovascular machine burns 3 times more calories than a standard treadmill. Restaurants promote foods for health conscious consumers such as low calorie, guiltless, low-carb, low-fat and under 500-calorie menu items.

Everywhere we look we are being told the key to weight loss is to reduce our calorie intake by eating less and exercising more.

Weight loss programs are focused on expending as many calories as possible. Even the fitness instructors on home workout DVD's and in group exercise classes cheer us on to *'feel the burn!'*

Fitness experts along with our own calorie consciousness tell us that exercise burns the most calories and therefore is the most important component of a weight loss program.

Today we have different resources available to track our calorie consumption and expenditure. Food labels tell us how many calories are in a certain product and even provide a list of the nutrients. There are calorie counting devices that compute the calories you burn during exercise. You can search the internet and find out how many calories specific activities and exercises burn. Even most cardiovascular exercise machines are now equipped with digital displays that read the number of calories burned during an exercise session.

However, a closer look seems to reveal that we've been secretly brainwashed.

I'm not saying this had been done on purpose but it's more of a case of the blind leading the blind.

Most calorie tracking devices only use a fraction of the information needed to accurately determine how many calories are expended during a workout.

There are many factors that determine how many calories you burn such as your age, weight, fitness level, muscle-to-fat ratio, stress level, hormones, external environment, internal and external temperature, hydration status and diet.

Determining many of these requires specialized equipment, strict testing procedures implemented by trained professionals and are typically performed in carefully controlled clinical settings.

Some of these factors can and do change on a daily basis. This means that the calories you burn during the same exercise or activity can change from one workout to the next making it nearly impossible to accurately determine the number of calories burned on a consistent basis.

Another point of consideration is that all calories are not equal and therefore how many calories you burn is not necessarily as important as where those calories come from.

For example, if you lose 10 pounds but 8 of those pounds come from protein, glycogen (carbohydrates that have been broken down and stored as a usable form of energy) and water the bulk of your weight loss came at the expense of lean body mass which slows down your metabolism making weight loss more difficult and weight rebound more likely.

As you have discovered throughout this book the current weight loss model of calorie expenditure has been oversimplified and is fundamentally flawed.

Burning calories for the sake of burning calories can be a recipe for disaster if those calories are not coming from the energy stored in your fat cells.

And, there's one deciding factor that ultimately determines where those calories come from...

...*that factor is stress.*

Stress can be categorized into 4 main types: mental, emotional, nutritional and physical.

In this chapter we'll be examining the effects of physical stress and why your body responds well to exercise some of the time and fights tooth and nail against it at other times and what you can do about it so losing weight is no longer a battle of wills between you and your body.

The Catch-22 Of Cardio

Cardiovascular exercise, commonly called *'cardio'*, has become the most popular and preferred form of physical stress for losing weight.

The popularity of cardio for weight loss came about somewhere in the 1980's after it was determined that cardiovascular exercise, which back then went by the name of *'aerobics'*, could help burn fat.

Today most health clubs house more cardio equipment than ever before. In addition to the typical treadmills, stationary bikes, stair climbers and elliptical machines, group exercise classes are growing in number and popularity. There are many options to choose from including step aerobics, cardio kick-boxing, salsa, zumba, spinning, sculpting and toning classes for just about every part of the body.

Many health clubs now have television sets displayed along the walls in the cardio area so club members can watch their favorite shows while peddling away on the stationary bike or strolling along the treadmill.

It seems America is crazy about cardio however cardio is not so crazy about America.

You'll find evidence of this in the cardio area of any health club by looking at the results of the *'regulars'*. Every health club has them and you can usually count them on one hand. By *'regulars'* I am referring to the few that seemingly spend every waking hour on their favorite cardio machine. You know who they are because every time you're there so are they. In fact, it's a good bet that if these cardioholics ever went missing they could be found in the cardio area at their local health club.

Why Cardio Is A Sucker's Bet

If you look around almost any health club you'll notice the most crowded area is the cardio area. Most people are using treadmills, stationary bikes, elliptical machines, stair steppers and participating in group exercise classes like step aerobics, cardio kick-boxing, spinning, water aerobics and other forms of cardiovascular exercise in an all-out effort to fight fat.

But, take a look around and ask yourself how many cardioholics have significantly changed their bodies with all that cardio over the last 3, 6 or 12 months. The answer is very few to none.

You would think that with the growing number of health club memberships and all of today's advanced technology producing better exercise equipment along with the growth and expansion of health clubs offering more group exercise classes we would see a significant decrease in the overweight population.

Instead, obesity is a nationwide epidemic that's on the rise.

Today we have more resources than ever on nutrition and exercise for weight loss as evidenced by the cluttered shelves in popular bookstores containing hundreds of diet and exercise books. We are constantly bombarded by television infomercials advertising *'miracle'* weight loss supplements, fad diets, tummy tightening and thigh slimming gadgets and gizmos.

Still the number of Americans who are overweight and obese continues to grow coupled with an alarming Increase in childhood obesity.

The reason why popular weight loss methods like cardio and diets are failing is because they only address the symptoms rather than the real cause of weight gain which is stress. I am not saying that cardiovascular fitness is unnecessary. It is an important component for optimum fitness and health but a lack of cardiovascular fitness it is not the <u>root cause</u> of our weight problems it is a <u>symptom</u>. Most people are trying all kinds of diets and doing so much cardio to lose weight only to see very little return on their *'investment'*.

In order to achieve lasting weight loss you must identify and eliminate the source of the problem. Eliminate the source and the symptoms will disappear.

The Shocking Truth About Cardio & Weight Loss

Before we get into the effects of too much physical stress let's take a look at the effectiveness of cardio for weight loss.

While the number of calories burned during exercise can look pretty outrageous they are also a bit misleading.

For example, statistics in the *ACE Personal Trainer Manual* reveal that an individual who weighs 170 pounds will burn approximately 13 calories per minute of running at a pace of 6 miles-per-hour.

Running at a 6 miles-per-hour pace is not a leisurely stroll along the beach, it's hard work for most people.

This equates to 780 calories burned per hour. However, an important fact is often overlooked. Not all of these calories are equal. If the bulk of your caloric expenditure comes from glycogen and protein and very little from fat you will ultimately break down muscle and slow your metabolism down.

Therefore the goal of an effective weight loss program is to maximize the utilization of fat for energy which, at best, is around 50%-60% of the total calories burned during a workout.

This means that at best about 60% of the 780 calories burned will come from fat. This equals 468 calories from fat.

One pound of fat is equal to 3,500 calories which means that at a body weight of 170 pounds it will take approximately **7 ½ hours to burn 1 pound of fat** at an expenditure of 60%. And, this does not factor in how many calories you put back through the foods consumed during the day which will *increase* the time it takes.

Even the excess post-exercise oxygen consumption (EPOC) known as the after-burn effect following exercise only contributes a maximum of slightly over 200 calories.

Considering work obligations and family commitments that demand so much of our time most of us have a difficult time squeezing just 3 hours of exercise into a typical week.

However, even managing 5 hours of exercise each week consisting of running at a 6 miles-per-hour pace it would take nearly two weeks to lose 1 pound of fat considering you actually eat on a daily basis.

A ratio of 2 weeks of exercise-to-1 pound of fat just doesn't seem like much of a return on your energy *'investment'* does it?

And, the lighter you are the longer it takes to burn that single pound of fat.

On the other hand, if you're thinking that since it takes a lighter person longer to burn a pound of fat then the opposite must be true you are correct. The heavier you are the less time it takes however; it is also more difficult to move a heavier body at the same intensity for the same length of time.

The final consideration is the energy requirements needed to maintain a 6 miles-per-hour pace for an entire hour. This level of intensity presents a significant challenge most people are unable to maintain for an entire hour let alone multiple times per week on a consistent basis.

Even if 100% of the calories burned came from fat (a physiological impossibility) it would still take 60 minutes of high-intensity exercise for nearly 5 days each week to lose one pound. How long do you think your body would hold up to this intensity?

High-intensity workouts are stressful to the body. If you are not completely recovered before the next onslaught you are adding stress on top of stress which eventually results in breakdown.

You can only perform so much high-intensity work before your body's capacity to handle the physical stress is compromised. Once this point is exceeded your body will do everything it can to conserve energy by breaking down muscle and slowing down your metabolism because it doesn't know whether you are working out like a maniac to lose weight or if you're stranded and starving in the middle of the Sahara desert. It's all stress.

This is one of the reasons why so many people who eat healthy and exercise all the time get stuck in a weight loss rut. They go 100% during every workout which accumulates until their capacity for physical stress is pushed over the limit.

They expend so much energy without enough going back in to the point where a large energy deficit is created and the body becomes overly stressed.

The body doesn't know it is not in any real danger because all stress is experienced in the same way. So, the body goes into energy conservation mode by doing everything it can to slow down energy expenditure.

This means that when a significant imbalance exists from too much physical stress even in the form of exercise the body can and will fight all of your efforts to lose weight. And, the more exercise you do or the harder you try only digs deeper into the already existing energy deficit to which your body resists.

The #1 Secret To Permanent Weight Loss & Optimum Health

When it comes to exercise we tend to think of our bodies much like an automobile...as a bunch of parts. It's really no surprise considering how much we are bombarded by the media.

We turn on our television sets and see *'Joey Washboard Abs'* showing how easy it is to crunch your way to a sexy stomach using the latest scientifically proven abdominal activation apparatus.

We flip through our favorite fitness magazines and see an ad by *'Suzy Slim Thighs'* promoting the fabulous wonder-glute gizmo that promises you a backside so firm you can bounce a quarter into a glass off of it.

However, when looking at the human body from a holistic perspective we are much more than just arms, thighs, abs, hips and calves. The human body is a system of integrated systems that all depend on each other.

That's why these body slimming gadgets fail to work. They are designed to target one area or part of the body. But, addressing one area without all the other important areas will not work.

For example, you will not lose excess belly fat by doing abdominal exercises alone. Belly fat is a symptom caused by poor nutrition, overeating, excess cortisol and inactivity.

So, if you want to know the #1 secret to lasting weight loss it's this…

…address the body as a whole rather than as individual parts.

Our bodies are a network of integrated systems including the cardiovascular (heart and blood vessels), musculoskeletal (muscles and bones), respiratory (lungs), integument (skin), lymphatic (immune), digestive (digestion), urinary (waste), nervous (nerves) and endocrine (hormones) systems.

All of these systems are different yet they work together. Creating a body that looks, feels and moves its' best is dependent upon balancing the system of systems that make up your body.

Many of my past clients were amazed at how, after years of being stuck at a certain body weight, they suddenly lost unwanted pounds and their nagging aches and pains disappeared by balancing these integrated systems without having to do hundreds of stomach squeezing sit-ups, painfully punishing push-ups or thigh thinning theatrics.

They didn't do long workouts nor spend every waking hour at the gym. They also ate **more** food rather than less. It was simply a matter of balancing the systems of the body thereby reducing stress.

All Exercise Is Not Created Equal

It's a known fact that losing weight and keeping it off requires exercise. Exercise is how we move energy throughout our bodies. However, just as exercising too little works against us, if we exercise too much our bodies become highly stressed and fight against our weight loss efforts.

The latter is a common theme among chronic over-exercisers who often perform rigorous workouts 5, 6 or even 7 days a week yet are unable to reach their weight loss goals even though many eat a healthy diet.

Achieving your weight loss goals requires proper management of your stress levels. Managing physical stress requires a balance between energy going out and energy coming into your body.

Exercise is typically associated with activities that use energy. We can call this *energy costing* exercise. Energy costing exercise is any exercise that causes your body to use more energy than it takes in.

Below are the 3 main types of energy costing exercise.

Types of Energy Costing Exercise

- Cardiovascular Exercise- Any form of activity that is maintained for a prolonged period of time (ex: 30 minutes) and presents some level of cardio respiratory challenge. Cardiovascular exercise improves the efficiency of the heart to pump blood, oxygen and nutrients throughout the body.

- Resistance Training- Any exercise that challenges the muscles of your body to work against resistance such as squats, push-ups, pull-ups, lunges, chest presses, overhead presses, rows, pulldowns and various other exercises. Too add variety you can perform many of these exercises with dumbbells, medicine balls, resistance bands or your own body weight. Resistance training provides several benefits such as improved muscular endurance, strength and/or power. Resistance training aids in weight loss through the addition or maintenance of lean body mass and by improving the efficiency of the working muscles to extract and use nutrients from the bloodstream such as glycogen and fatty acids as energy. Resistance training also conditions the muscular system to increase its' work capacity and thus handle increased levels of physical stress.

- <u>Sports Activities</u>- Any sport such as tennis, running, basketball, soccer, softball, volleyball and others. Most sporting activities involve a combination of cardiovascular and resistance training.

This is where it is important to understand the concept of your stress threshold. If you are stressed to the point that you are over your threshold any more stress will be detrimental. This means performing an intense energy costing workout when you are over your stress threshold will do more harm than good.

Remember, piling stress on top of a system that's overwhelmed from stress will eventually break it down while making weight loss a virtually unwinnable battle.

For this purpose there are alternative types of exercise for effectively reducing physical stress and cultivating energy within the body that can help rejuvenate a sluggish metabolism and get your weight loss back on track. These are *energy building* exercises.

Energy building exercises can be used on days between regular energy costing workouts or whenever you feel emotionally, mentally or physically stressed.

An energy building exercise is any exercise that helps your body take in more energy than it uses. This is a key concept because your body needs energy to use energy. Think of your body like your car and energy like gasoline. If you want your car to operate it needs gasoline. If all you do is drive your car from one destination to another you'll use up all the gas. So, you fill your tank up with gas to keep your car running because your car needs gasoline in order to use gasoline.

Our bodies function in a very similar way in that they need energy to use energy. Energy building exercise helps produce energy, promotes recovery, energy balance and energy flow; all of which are needed for stress reduction that leads to weight loss, health and vitality.

How To Overcome Nagging Aches and Pains

Approximately 70% of non-contact injuries are caused by muscle imbalances. Many of our daily activities involve repetitive movements and postures that cause certain muscles to become short and tight while others become long and weak. These muscle imbalances increase wear and tear on our muscles and joints, create poor posture, restrict blood and energy flow, inhibit weight loss and contribute to those nagging aches and pains we often blame on old age.

A former client of mine came to me after surgeries and exercise failed to relieve her physical pain. She wanted to give exercise one last chance to help relive the chronic pain that had taken over her life. She was in her early 50's and suffered from degenerative disk disease that had her bed-ridden most of her days, taking a number of medications and a 5 pound lifting limit.

Although her condition could not be reversed, I believed the effects could be delayed as long as possible by correcting her existing muscle imbalances that were causing stress to her lower back where most of her pain originated from.

Within 6 months she showed amazing improvement and within 3 years she was a completely different person.

I'll let you read it in her own words:

"One year after wondering if I would ever be able to walk again unaided I am confidently planning to do 40 miles in 2 days for a charity walk. My everyday activities have increased and most days I can do more than I ever thought I could before I started my training."

She also dropped 4 clothing sizes and added 10 pounds of lean muscle.

It was just a matter of retraining her body to move more efficiently that reduced the overall physical stress she was dealing with and got her looking, feeling and moving better than she had in years.

The way to overcome those nagging aches and pains is to consume a diet high in nutrients and to correct your muscle imbalances.

For over 10 years I have witnessed patients I worked with, my own clients, friends and family members successfully overcome neck, shoulder, lower back, hip, knee, ankle and foot problems that had plagued them for so long by following this simple approach.

6 Powerful Energy Building Methods To Rejuvenate Body & Mind

The methods listed below do not represent the only energy building methods and are meant to serve as a starting point.

- Yoga- An ancient Indian body of knowledge consisting of exercises and breathing techniques focused on improving flexibility, circulation and increasing awareness of the body and mind to help relieve stress.

- Stretching- If you are flexible then you probably don't mind stretching. However, if you are inflexible then you can probably think of just about anything you would rather do than stretch. Stretching offers more than just a quick warm-up prior to a workout.

There are a number of stretching methods that can help restore muscle balance, joint alignment, posture and energy flow that go beyond the purpose of this book.

However, here are some simple guidelines for stretching:

1. Be sure the muscles are properly warmed up prior to stretching. Performing 8-10 minutes of light

activity such as walking or biking is usually sufficient.

2. Stretch immediately after exercise since the muscles are thoroughly warm and can be easily stretched.

3. Hold each stretch for 10-30 seconds.

4. Stretch only those muscles that feel tight or restricted. If you do not feel anything when stretching a muscle it may not need stretching.

- <u>Massage</u>- Massage therapy produces many physiological and psychological benefits such as increased relaxation, circulation, energy, quality of sleep, recovery and concentration along with decreased anxiety, fatigue and stress.

There are many different types of massage available and a little research can help you determine which is right for you. You can also contact a licensed massage therapist in your area to learn more.

- <u>Polarity Therapy</u>- A natural health care system that works with energy fields that exist is the human body. According to the polarity model pain and disease arise when energy is unbalanced, blocked or fixed due to stress or other factors. This may work from a weight loss standpoint as well since losing weight requires efficient energy movement.

Stress creates tension in the muscles. When the muscles are constantly tense blood, oxygen and nutrients cannot properly circulate throughout the body which can negatively affect the energy supply to muscles, organs and other tissues.

A polarity therapy session is performed by a trained practitioner and is designed to balance energy flow through soft touch, light rocking and point specific touch.

You can find out more information on Polarity Therapy at the *American Polarity Therapy Association's* website: http://www.polaritytherapy.org

- Tai-Chi- An ancient Chinese form of movement focused on cultivating energy within the body. Tai Chi is used to harmonize the mind, body and spirit while promoting physical and mental well being.

If practiced consistently energy can efficiently move throughout the body providing strength against the stresses from our environment, our food and our *'on-the-go'* lifestyles.

- Meditation- Because we live highly stressful lives tension builds up within our bodies and breathing often becomes shallow and restricted which reduces the amount of oxygen (*and energy*) available within the body. Think of how you feel when you get really stressed out. Your muscles get tense, you become more rigid and you take in less oxygen. Oxygen is what gives us life sustaining energy and when we take in less of it we have less energy available.

Meditation helps relax the body and mind and improve physical, mental, emotional and spiritual well-being. Many forms of meditation involve deep, slow, relaxed breathing which brings energy into the body by taking in more oxygen. Oxygen is transported through the bloodstream from the lungs to the heart where it is pumped to all parts of the body and plays a critical role in the energy building process.

Energy building methods are vital for stress management and weight loss. They are needed to balance energy going out of the body with energy coming in yet are often overlooked particularly when it comes to exercise.

This is because we tend to associate exercise only with a loss of energy or *'working out'*. When energy going out becomes significantly greater than energy coming in an imbalance is created within the body. If this imbalance becomes too great the body eventually becomes overly stressed, resistant to weight loss and more susceptible to injury, sickness and disease.

We live in very stressful times where we are on the go from the time we wake up until the time our head hits the pillow. Most of our energy reserves are depleted during our day and then we wonder why we find it so difficult to fit exercise into our lives.

We're trying to combat a lack of energy by using more energy without putting enough of it back in the tank.

If your goal is to lose weight, have more energy and build optimal health it is critical to balance the physical stress of working *out* with working *in*.

The Key To Managing Physical Stress For Lasting Weight Loss

Brief periods of sympathetic nervous system (SNS) activity are beneficial and healthy. Exercise activates the SNS which triggers the release of glucocorticoids, catecholamines, blood glucose and fatty acids for energy production.

When SNS activity stays below your threshold for stress it helps trigger the parasympathetic nervous system (PNS) which is your body's recovery or rebuilding system. PNS activity stimulates digestion and metabolism as well as the release of tissue building hormones such as growth hormone, DHEA and testosterone which help to maintain and build lean muscle and burn fat. When both systems are balanced you will experience increased energy, optimal responses to exercise and better recovery from exercise and other stressors.

Too much physical stress results in SNS dominance, muscle breakdown, decreased recovery and increased fat storage. The following are warning signs indicating you may have exceeded your capacity for physical stress:

- Increased heart rate or blood pressure
- Increased mental, physical or emotional fatigue
- Sickness and infection
- Poor quality of sleep
- Decreased desire to exercise
- Decreased mental or physical performance
- Irritability or mood swings
- Decreased strength or stamina

If you experience one or more of these warning signs it is best to take some time off from energy costing activities and include energy building exercises to allow the appropriate recovery to take place.

Too little physical stress results in PNS dominance which can be good if your body is overworked and needs some down time. However, when completely recovered, a PNS dominant state can be detrimental toward weight loss and optimum health due to the lack of energy movement throughout the body.

The key to managing physical stress for weight loss, health and well being is balancing the energy costing sympathetic nervous system with the energy building parasympathetic nervous system.

The balance of energy costing and energy building exercise provides a simple, effective way to use physical activity to keep your stress levels balanced while losing weight.

Conclusion

The solution to better health and weight loss is simple but not easy. I hope this book has helped you gain a better understanding of how you can lose weight, reduce body fat and improve your health by reducing the 4 main stressors that are responsible for weight problems, sickness and disease.

My purpose for writing this book is to help empower 1 million people worldwide to achieve permanent weight loss, health and fitness.

Fad diets, weight loss pills, supplements and body toning machines come and go just as sure as the sun will rise tomorrow. By using the principles in this book you will never need to depend on ineffective weight loss strategies that only work for a short time and then stop leaving you frustrated and confused as you search for the next *'solution'*.

You will never need to count another calorie, weigh or measure foods or tally up points—that is unless you want to. Nor will you ever need to resort to extreme and unhealthy fad diets, bogus weight loss supplements or the latest body toning gimmicks advertised on late night television infomercials and magazine ads.

That's the beauty of using principles rather than strategies. Strategies are always changing because they don't work for everyone or for very long (if at all). Principles on the other hand work over the long-term and never change because they don't need to.

This book contains the exact blueprint you need to successfully reach your weight loss goals and create the body you want. One that not only looks good on the outside but feels and functions just as well on the inside.

Your road to a leaner, firmer and more attractive body begins now.

Enjoy the journey.

Best wishes,

Kevin Yates

P.S. I would like to take this time to ask you to help me achieve my goal of helping 1 million people achieve their weight loss and fitness goals by forwarding a copy of this book to everyone you know of who needs it.

An even better idea is to order hard copy versions to give away as gifts to those who will greatly benefit from the information in this book.

With your help we can create miracles!

About The Author

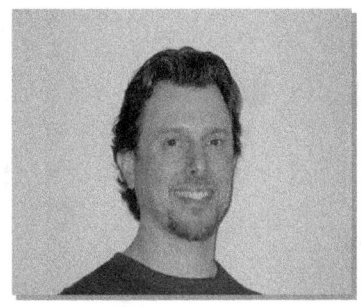 Kevin Yates is a holistic health expert, speaker and author who has empowered people to overcome the mental and physical obstacles to achieve their health and fitness goals for over 11 years.

Kevin believes that optimum health is a balance between mental, emotional, nutritional and physical health that is best achieved by training both the body and mind through a holistic approach integrating principles of nutrition and exercise, personal growth and development, success and achievement and mindset and motivation.

Kevin currently teaches workshops and seminars for business owners, companies and their staff on how to lower stress and improve health so they can effectively reduce work related stress, improve focus and productivity and decrease missed work time.

Kevin lives in Lathrop, California with his wife of 11 years Veronica and their 4 year-old daughter Briana.

If you are interested in booking Kevin to speak at your event please contact him at:
kyates@yatesperformancetraining.com or
http://thestressfreediet.com

Resources:

How To Eat, Move and Be Healthy, 2004. Paul Chek.

The Last 4 Doctors You'll Ever Need, Paul Chek.

Eat Stop Eat, 2010. Brad Pilon. pg. 90

How Much Protein, 2011. Brad Pilon

The Elimination Diet, 2010, Dax Moy. pg. 76

The Diet Solution, 2009. Isabel De Los Rios. pg. 58

Thresholds Of The Mind, 2007. Bill Harris. pg. 69

The Divine Matrix, 2007. Gregg Braden.

Energy Medicine, 1998. Donna Eden with David Feinstein, Ph.D pg. 40

The Spontaneous Healing Of Belief, 2008. Gregg Braden pp.43-44

The Skinny On Fats, 1999. Mary Enig, Ph.D and Sally Fallon. pg. 3

ACE Personal Trainer Manual, 2003. American Council On Exercise. pg. 231